W9-CMB-915

IBS:

A Doctor's Plan for
Chronic Digestive Troubles

THE DEFINITIVE GUIDE to PREVENTION & RELIEF

IBS:

A Doctor's Plan for Chronic Digestive Troubles

THE DEFINITIVE GUIDE to PREVENTION & RELIEF

Third Edition
Revised & Enlarged

GERARD GUILLORY, M.D.

Hartley
&Marks
PUBLISHERS

Published by
HARTLEY & MARKS PUBLISHERS INC.
P. O. Box 147   3661 West Broadway
Point Roberts, WA   Vancouver, BC
98281   V6R 2B8

Design and composition by The Typeworks
Set in Stone Serif

Printed in the U.S.A.

LIBRARY OF CONGRESS CATALOGING-IN-PUBLICATION DATA

Guillory, Gerard.
    IBS : a doctor's plan for chronic digestive troubles : the defintive guide
to prevention and relief / Gerard Guillory.—3rd ed.
    p. cm.
    Includes index.
    ISBN 0-88179-179-2
    1. Irritable colon.   I. Title.

RC862.I77 G85 2001
616.3'44—dc 21   2001024135

NOTICE TO THE READER

This book is meant to be a source of information for those who are interested in learning about IBS, including mechanisms and methods. Every person has different health problems and issues, based on age, gender, lifestyle, health status, genetics, diet, psychological state, and spiritual maturity. My intent is to share my experience and offer guidelines to help you become more informed about your healthcare choices and options. In cooperation with your physician and other healthcare providers, you can then take the necessary steps to maintain optimum health. This book is sold with the understanding that the publisher is not engaged in rendering medical or other professional services. If medical or expert assistance is required, the services of a competent professional should be sought. Neither the author nor the publisher takes medical or legal responsibility for the reader who uses the contents of this book as a prescription.

Man should always strive to have his intestines relaxed all the days of his life.

— Maimonides, *12th century physician*

The word "doctor" has its roots in the Latin word meaning "to teach," and patient education is an important aspect of the healing arts. As stated in the *American College of Physicians Ethos Manual:* "The patient should be informed and educated about his condition and should understand and approve of the treatment. In return, he should participate responsibly in his own care."

Table of Contents

Foreword to the Third Edition

Iᴠ ʏᴏᴜ ᴏʀ ꜱᴏᴍᴇᴏɴᴇ you are close to is afflicted by IBS, then you know the toll it can take. You may also appreciate that IBS is poorly understood. Fortunately, increased research into this area has led to significant advances in our understanding of this complex disorder. For example, in our body their exists an extensive network of neurons that communicate between the brain and the gut. This brain-gut, bidirectional connection processes information in such a way that our emotions may affect our digestion and the digestive processes may affect how we feel.

We often express ourselves in relation to our "viscera", our internal organs. "What's your gut reaction?", "Go with your gut instinct!", "You make me sick to my stomach". Physicians in the past were told that IBS was a "functional disorder" and patients were often made to feel that the symptoms were "all in your head". Uncertainty about the diagnosis often led to more testing which further fueled anxiety about what might really be wrong.

Now the diagnosis of IBS can be made with confidence in collaboration with your physician after a detailed history and appropriate studies. It is no longer considered a "diagnosis of exclusion". Treatment begins with patient education. And patient education begins with a discussion of our current understanding of the underlying abnormalities which produce IBS symptoms.

IBS is a disorder wherein there is a problem between the brain and the enteric nervous system or so-called "gut brain" connection. With IBS, the "wiring"— the neurons that control motility, secretion, and the perception of pain in the intestinal tract—is not regulated properly, making IBS a disorder of function. IBS sufferers experience a heightened perception of pain in the gut referred to as "visceral hypersensitivity". Various substances, referred to as neurotransmitters such as serotonin, may play an important role with regard to gut function. Our emotions, our diet and hormones may all adversely impact IBS. When our gut doesn't function well, we can't function well and the impact on our quality of life can be significant.

It is estimated that up to 20% of the population may suffer with IBS. Although it is felt to be more common in women, up to 5% of men in the U. S. also suffer from IBS. IBS may contribute to the "corporate glass ceiling" because many affected women have refused promotions, refused to travel, cut back on their hours, worked from home, have changed or lost their jobs as a result of uncontrolled IBS symptoms.

As a gastroenterologist, I have treated many patients suffering from IBS over the years. Imagine my delight when I began to read Dr. Guillory's book and found honest, personal, up-to-date, and accurate advice from cover to cover. Understanding irritable bowel syndrome and learning how to control it gives us power. Dr. Guillory's book clearly outlines many strategies that doctors and patients can take to improve the health and function of those suffering from IBS. This reliable source of information addresses the issues that IBS patients face in an insightful, intelligent, and compassionate manner.

Christine Frissora, M.D., F.A.C.P.
Assistant Professor of Medicine
Weill Cornell Medical Center
New York Presbyterian Hospital

Foreword to the First Edition

IT IS MY BELIEF that Dr. Guillory has provided an important source of reference information for patients. The term "doctor" actually means teacher, derived from the Latin term "docere"—to teach. Teaching for and to medical students as they study to become physicians and continuing medical education for physicians in practice is a well-recognized teaching goal. Teaching patients to understand the principles of good health and to deal with health problems intelligently is, in my view, an equally important responsibility for the physician and is one which has not been as well met by the medical profession. And while other members of the health care team, nutritionists, pharmacists and nurse practitioners can help with patient education, the ultimate responsibility lies with the physician.

In the "good old days," physicians were apt to deal with patient concerns and questions in a paternalistic, sometimes patronizing fashion, leaving the patient with unanswered questions and anxieties, even though frequently the patient's problem was eventually "cured." No more! We live in an age of consumer activism. In medicine, patients want and frequently demand (rightly so) to know what the physician thinks might be wrong, what tests are being done and why, and what therapy is to be employed, and what options exist. Modern medicine has made remarkable strides in dealing with problems and diseases; much of the success has resulted from the application of complex technology both in the diagnosis and treatment of disease. Not only must physicians understand the application of these technologies, they must be able and willing to determine that the patient understands as well. Decisions concerning diagnosis and treatment require patient participation, and patients can intelligently participate only if they understand the issues involved. There are several ways in which patients can learn more and therefore make appropriate decisions. One of those ways is through the availability of written material done from the lay person's perspective and exemplified in Dr. Guillory's book. I would stress, however, that such material is intended only to complement patient understanding and should never be used as a guide to self-treatment or to replace appropriate medical care.

Of all the patient complaints seen by primary care physicians, those related to the gastrointestinal tract are the most common and amongst these, irritable bowel syndrome (IBS) is an especially important problem. As Dr. Guillory points out, the diagnosis of this problem is one of exclusion; there is no specific diagnostic test which confirms the diagnosis, so the physician relies on a careful history and the appropriate use of studies to exclude other, sometimes more serious disorders which can mimic IBS. The book is primarily intended for the intelligent lay reader and is written in an informal, though not patronizing style. You can literally feel the author's desire to help patients understand this perplexing problem. He begins with the definition of IBS and leads the reader through many possible causes, or factors, which may aggravate symptoms, emphasizing diet and emotions, and then discusses all aspects of the symptomatic treatment of the disease.

Of special value are the sections on other common gastrointestinal diseases which mimic IBS, and the diagnostic studies which may be required to exclude other diseases. The useful glossary explains much of the medical jargon in understandable terms. My hope is that patients who read this book will receive hope and encouragement about management of the condition and that physicians will use it, and material like it, as they educate patients about the disease.

O'Neill Barrett, Jr, MD.
Professor Emeritus
Department of Medicine
University of South Carolina
School of Medicine

Acknowledgments

ALTHOUGH IT IS customary to acknowledge those who have contributed to an author's work, I do so with some trepidation as it is impossible to thank everyone who deserves my gratitude for this third edition of *IBS: A Doctor's Plan for Chronic Digestive Troubles.*

I would like to thank the many patients I have treated over the years who have helped me understand the complexities of IBS and the difficulties associated with experiencing IBS. I would like to thank my wife Cheryll, a former IBS sufferer who was a catalyst for fostering my interest in IBS almost 20 years ago.

I would also like to thank the many physician colleagues with whom I work and those practitioners who share an interest in treating patients with functional gastrointestinal disorders. A special thanks to Dr. Paul Donovan for his contribution to this edition as well as the last. Thanks to Dr. Vanessa Ameen, Dr. Raphael d'Angelo, Dr. Jack Martin, and Matt Vogl for their contributions to this edition.

Lastly thanks to Sharon McCann and the editiorial staff at Hartley & Marks for their support and patience.

About the Author and Contributors

The Author

GERARD GUILLORY, M.D. is an internist in private practice in Aurora, Colorado, and also an assistant clinical professor at the University of Colorado Health Sciences Center. He has had a long-standing interest in IBS and gives frequent lectures to both medical audiences and the general public on this topic. His wife of 18 years, a former IBS sufferer, served as a catalyst for development of his interest in this area. A diplomat of the American Board of Internal Medicine, he has prepared numerous public education materials. He stresses the value of patient participation and responsibility in treatment, and the importance of lifestyle changes in all treatment programs.

The Contributors

VANESSA Z. AMEEN, M.D. is a board-certified pediatric gastroenterologist with over 15 years experience in academic and clinical medicine and the pharmaceutical industry. Over the years, she has been engaged in patient care, teaching, clinical research, and administration of pediatric gastroenterology and nutrition programs. Dr. Ameen was a technical advisor to the Working Group on Functional GI Disorders for the First World Congress of Pediatric Gastroenterology, Hepatology and Nutrition, and is a member of several professional societies. She frequently speaks to health care professionals about gastroenterology, nutrition, and clinical research and practice.

RAPHAEL J. D'ANGELO, M.D. is a board-certified holistic family physician in Aurora, Colorado, and is an assistant clinical professor of family practice at the University of Colorado Health Sciences Center. He received his medical degree from the University of Oklahoma in 1976 and served in the U.S. Air Force as a family physician and allergist until entering private practice in 1982. A member of the American Holistic Medical Association and a certified aromatherapist, he has written extensively on complementary and alternative medicine topics and gives talks and seminars to health professionals and the public.

PAUL B. DONOVAN, Ph.D. is a clinical psychophysiologist and director of a clinic in Santa Fe, New Mexico. A specialist in the treatment of chronic functional disorders, Dr. Donovan has developed patient self-management programs for functional disorders of the gastrointestinal, musculo-skeletal, and cardiovascular systems. He is a member of the medical advisory board of the International Foundation for Functional Gastrointestinal Disorders, and is a sought-after speaker for IBS associations in several countries. Dr. Donovan received his Ph.D. from the University of Queensland, Australia.

JACK MARTIN, Ph.D. has a private practice in stress management and psychotherapy with offices in Aurora and Estes Park, Colorado as well as Corpus Christi, Texas. Dr. Martin specializes in working with people who have stress-related physical problems such as IBS. His certifications from professional organizations include the American Academy of Pain Management, the Biofeedback Certification Institute of America, the American Association of Psychophysiology and Biofeedback, the American Academy of Sleep Medicine, and the American Board of Medical Psychotherapists.

MATT VOGL is a stand-up comedian working in Colorado and other Western states. He balances his comedy with a job in public health, helping communities set up nurse home visiting programs. His humorous short stories grew out of his stage comedy, and he is currently at work on a collection of short stories based on his experiences. Matt resides in Denver, Colorado with his wife, Sarah.

Preface

IF YOU ARE ONE in five adults in North America, the chances are that you have or know someone who has irritable bowel syndrome (IBS). An estimated 20 percent of the population in the U.S. have this common gastrointestinal disorder, which can last a lifetime. If you do have IBS, the chances are also that you were alarmed and frustrated when told that there is no cure. Due to the nature of the symptoms, IBS can be a socially isolating disorder. For this reason, I included "One Patient's Experience of IBS" by Matt Vogl as the introduction to the third edition of this book.

Matt Vogl shares with humor his painful (and perhaps common) experience of how he and his doctor arrived at the diagnosis of IBS. Traditionally, a diagnosis of IBS was made by a process of exclusion and exhaustive testing. Not only were the tests costly and time-consuming, but they also left IBS sufferers with the feeling that no one was sure about what they had.

Today, there remains no single conclusive test to diagnose IBS. However, in the last four years since the previous edition of this book, significant progress has been made in the diagnosis and treatment of IBS. In 1999, the Rome II criteria were published, making it easier for physicians to diagnose IBS using a clear set of guidelines. Ongoing research into the connections between the central nervous system and the enteric nervous system is explaining why many IBS sufferers have increased visceral sensitivity.

In response to a growing interest in complementary alternative medicine (CAM), I have included a new chapter and section on CAM therapies used to treat IBS. Just as it is true of traditional medicine, alternative medicine needs ongoing evidence-based research to become a reliable foundation for diagnosis and treatment. To provide readers with the most authoritative information currently available on CAM therapies, I have gone to reliable sources. Dr. Raphael d'Angelo is a family physician and member of the American Holistic Medical Association who teaches at the University of Colorado Medical School. He has contributed a new chapter on the role of vitamins, herbs, beneficial bacteria, and digestive enzymes in the holistic treatment of IBS. Dr. Jack Martin, a psychotherapist who specializes in stress management, has also contributed a section on biofeedback and updated the chapter, "Stress and the Intestinal Tract." He explains how biofeedback works to alter physiologic functions and relieve associated symptoms of IBS. Biofeedback is most effective when used in combination with stress management techniques, which are also discussed in this chapter.

I am also pleased to include a new chapter written by Dr. Paul Donovan, a psychophysiologist who specializes in the treatment of functional disorders such as IBS. In "Understanding the Psychophysiology of IBS," Dr. Donovan explains how your body reacts to thoughts, feelings, and daily circumstances and affects the neurological regulation of the gastrointestinal tract. He explains the benefits of cognitive behavioral therapy—a four-step method of information control, cognitive control, behavioral control, and autonomic control.

This comprehensive and authoritative third edition would not be complete without a chapter on IBS in children and adolescents. Dr. Vanessa Ameen, a pediatric gastroenterologist, has written a chapter to help parents identify and cope with functional GI disorders in children and adolescents. She explains that while some of these disorders accompany normal development, others can significantly interfere with it. An important section for parents is how to recognize and manage functional abdominal pain, a common, often challenging childhood GI disorder for parents and physicians alike.

I truly hope this book helps you to understand the multiple causes and treatments of a complex disorder. I first began writing patient-education materials when I was a medical student. Over 15 years as a specialist in internal medicine and frequent lecturer about IBS, I have remained committed to health education. From experience I know that when you are fully informed about your ailment, you will be much more likely to participate in your healing, and become free of symptoms that need not affect your quality of life.

Gerard Guillory, M.D.
Aurora, Colorado

One Patient's Experience of IBS

by Matt Vogl

W<small>HEN I WAS</small> in elementary school I used to get teased a lot by the school bullies. I'm not sure why they teased me. Maybe it was the fact that I was skinny and weighed less than many toddlers. Maybe it was my thick Bob Griese glasses, or maybe it was the fact that teachers called on me more than other kids. Whatever the reason, they teased me. When I would come home crying to my mom about the way the other kids treated me, she said, "Just laugh at them." Thinking that this would only lead to getting beat up, I asked her to explain. She told me that if I laughed when they teased me, I was no longer giving them power over me, and it would remind me not to take their words so literally. I tried it, and it worked. Humor, I learned, has incredible disarming power.

Everyone has their own approach for dealing with the emotional and psychological aspects of irritable bowel syndrome (IBS). Some choose to attend support groups, some meditate, and some turn to exercise. As a freelance writer and amateur comedian, I have found that one of the ways I cope with stressful situations is by trying to find humor in them. Like my mother said, finding things to laugh at in a situation is a way of not letting something external have power over me. If the success of the movie *Patch Adams* is any indication, the use of humor is gaining acceptance in health care like never before.

In 1999 I was diagnosed with IBS and began working with Dr. Guillory to treat it. He gave me a copy of his book, *IBS: A Doctor's Plan for Chronic Digestive Troubles,* which helped me to better understand IBS. I hadn't known that some sufferers actually have the opposite of my problem: constipation. Must be nice, I thought.

Like so many others who suffer from IBS, I found the experience of trying to find out what was wrong with me to be incredibly frustrating and aggravating. I was embarrassed by how often I had to excuse myself to go to the bathroom and angry at the fact that the attacks inevitably came at the most inopportune moments. I tried and failed at the process of self-diagnosis, and finally sought the help of a physician after a particularly bad incident at work.

The process of working with a doctor to find out what was wrong with me was embarrassing, awkward, uncomfortable, and even humiliating at times. But ultimately I benefited because I finally had a name for what was wrong with me. IBS is a tough diagnosis to take because there is no cure, but as awareness and understanding increase, new approaches to dealing with it seem to be available every day.

One of the things that I've found most frustrating about IBS is that people are uncomfortable talking about it, so it can be extremely isolating for those who have it. I mean, who wants to talk to their friends about their bowel movements? But what's ironic is that the experience of IBS is almost universal: One in five people has IBS, and realistically, everybody else has experienced IBS-type symptoms at one time or another.

When I looked back on experiences I have suffered due to IBS, I realized that many of the events and interactions were humorous. I found that by focusing on the humorous aspects of my IBS, I was able to talk about it more. I told my friends the stories about being stuck in traffic and wondering if I would make it to a rest stop. And I told them about times I came home running into my house, leaving the car door open and running past my family without saying anything to make it to the bathroom in the nick of time. I noticed something about my friends' reactions to these stories: More often than not they would laugh, and then shyly admit that something like that had happened to them, which opened an opportunity to talk about it. It is incredibly comforting to know you are not alone in experiencing these things, and being able to laugh at aspects of my IBS has given me a certain power and freedom over the condition that I did not have before.

I wrote "There's a Bomb in the Building" to chronicle my struggles with IBS, my fear of physicians, and the frustrating process of trying to find out why I had to go to the bathroom all the time. I chose to highlight the humor in my own condition as a way to give other people permission to laugh at some of their own experiences with IBS. While the story is personal, people who have read it often say "That exact thing happened to me" and are then able to laugh about it.

Don't get me wrong—I don't think IBS is entirely a laughing matter. It is a serious condition that causes countless people, including myself, extreme discomfort. When you are having an episode, there is nothing funny about it at the time, but finding some humor in those situations helps to lighten the discomfort. I think of IBS as one of the playground bullies who teased me as a kid, and humor is still the best way I've found for not giving that bully too much power over me.

There's a Bomb in the Building

"There's a bomb in the building. You have two minutes."

Click. Dial tone.

The secretary receiving the bomb threat was new to the company. They had talked about bomb threats during her orientation, but she didn't pay attention. "Nobody really gets bomb threats," she had thought. The company seemed to have a policy for just about everything: things like bomb threats, hurricanes, hostage situations, volcanic eruptions, employee shootings, earthquakes, alien invasions, Soviet attacks, and all sorts of other things she was sure would never happen. Now, frantically fumbling through her "Policy and Procedures" manual she wished she had paid attention. Finding the section on bomb threats, she quickly scanned the page: "In case of a bomb threat it is imperative to keep the caller on the line as long as possible." Tossing the manual aside, she grabbed the phone and anxiously dialed building security. "Some guy just called," she stuttered. "He, he said there was a bomb and we have only two minutes!"

There are no negotiations during a bomb threat. The caller tells you how much time you have and hangs up. That's it. You don't ask for another minute or two, and there is no chance to negotiate the terms. If the caller says two minutes, then you have two minutes.

Your body talks to you. Your brain constantly sends messages asking you to consider certain courses of action. Usually, it just offers casual suggestions like "You know, I could go for a cheeseburger right about now," or "Hey, left leg itches. Scratch the left leg," or "Gosh this pavement is hot. Maybe you need shoes." But sometimes, when you are sick, your body speaks with the urgency of a bomb threat. In these situations there is no warning, no room for negotiation, and no asking for more time.

"There is a bomb in your body: you have diarrhea. You have two minutes to find a bathroom."

Click. Dial tone.

The sudden, sharp and stabbing abdominal pain and the dread that total loss of bowel control is imminent are the worst feelings a person can have. Everyone has experienced it at one time or another, but few people talk about it. As the contractions in your belly become more frequent and severe, you know that a violent release is inevitable, and nothing will slow it. Your body pleads with you to take the warning seriously, because failure to do so invites the most disastrous and embarrassing consequences. It never seems to happen when you are conveniently near a bathroom with nothing else to do. It is like your body is playing a practical joke on you, which invariably happens at the worst possible times: in meetings, on blind dates, on airplanes, on a ski chair lift, when camping, or when sitting in your car in rush hour traffic. Unfortunately, last summer it was happening to me with alarming frequency.

I knew something was very wrong with me when the routine call of nature became something more like a frantic primal scream almost on a daily basis. In just one week, I had to abruptly excuse myself and leave a job interview because I had sudden diarrhea. I returned sweating and embarrassed, only to find out I didn't get the job. After work the next day it happened again while hiking in the woods near my house. I had to relieve myself in a hastily dug latrine with only a pine cone to clean up with. Two days later when driving to meet a friend for lunch, I had to suddenly pull my car over at a construction site and beg a group of snickering carpenters to let me use their port-a-potty.

"What is happening to me?" I thought. "Do I have the flu? Salmonella? Did I eat bad cheese?" I kept thinking it would just go away; hoping it would go away, but it didn't. Diarrhea was becoming a daily occurrence. After three weeks of using the bathroom nine or ten times a day, I was weak and dehydrated. I accepted the fact that I was not getting any better and that I had to do something about it.

I've never liked going to the doctor. I'm intimidated by the fact that they know more about my body than I do. To me, doctors are kind of like car mechanics. A mechanic could tell me I need new muffler bearings and I would pay him a thousand dollars to replace them. If a doctor told me I needed a digestive system transplant, I would probably believe him because he knows more about it than I do. But at least when you go to a mechanic, you get to keep your clothes on.

It seems like the doctors I've gone to always want me to take off my clothes before they talk about diet or blood pressure. I'm self-conscious about my body and I don't like to undress in front of people I don't know. I am one of those people who wears a t-shirt in public swimming pools so other people won't see my chest, so I couldn't imagine sitting in my underwear and chatting with a fully clothed stranger about my bowel movements. I do anything to avoid going to doctors and as a result, tend to live in medical denial. "This tumor on my neck? Oh, that's nothing. It will go away, I'm sure." I pretend that cavities will heal themselves so I don't have to go to a dentist. "I can just chew on the other side," I reason. For ten years I ignored painful ingrown toenails because the thought of someone picking at my naked feet made me hyperventilate. I knew that if I went to a doctor about chronic diarrhea, I would have to answer a zillion questions and he would want to examine the scene of the crimes. Toes were bad enough; an examination of my rear end was completely out of the question. I wouldn't see a doctor, so I turned to my friends instead.

It is strange talking to family and friends about diarrhea. I felt dirty, as if what was wrong with me was as much about character as biology. Telling people you have chronic diarrhea feels like admitting that you are a drug addict or something. People are comfortable talking about headaches, cancer, high cholesterol, and all kinds of other ailments; but most are initially uncomfortable talking about digestive problems. But I found that once I brought it up, everybody had a story to tell and an opinion to share. Everybody either knew someone who had the same problem or had once experienced the same thing themselves.

"You eat too much cheese," my friend Stacy told me. "My aunt had the same deal. Lactose intolerance or something like that. She had to go to the bathroom all the time. It was bad. She finally wound up in the hospital after eating a bunch of pizza and ice cream one night. The doctors said she was allergic to dairy products and now she can't eat ice cream or cheese or any of that stuff."

My friend Marci is a glass-half-empty kind of person who gets overly dramatic and pessimistic about everything, but she was a nurse for ten years, which made her the closest thing to an expert among my friends, so I called her. I told her what was happening to me and she said I probably had cancer. She explained that colon cancer is really dangerous and a lot of people go for years ignoring the obvious symptoms until it is too late. "You may think you just have a bad case of the runs, but that cramping and the diarrhea you have are sure signs of colon cancer," she said. "Got blood in your stools? Because if there is, then it's probably too late. Seriously, you should go see a doctor about it. Tons of people die from that, you know. I'm not kidding. Don't screw around with cancer. I know of at least three people who ignored the warning signs of cancer and you know where they are now? Dead, that's where. Dead, dead, dead. I'm serious, Matt. Don't. Screw. With. Cancer."

"Crohn's disease for sure," was my brother Mark's opinion. "They're not really sure what causes it or how to cure it, but you have all the symptoms. I read something about it in *People* magazine. Ted Danson or Sting or somebody like that had it. They put you on really a bland high-fiber diet and you can't eat anything spicy or drink beer at all. But it sounds like Crohn's for sure. That or stress. Or cancer. One of those. Who the hell knows what you have? You think I'm a doctor? Glad it's not me, though. I know a guy at work who gets wicked diarrhea anytime he has to give a presentation because public speaking makes him so nervous. Maybe you just have bad nerves. Wife stressing you out? You really nervous about something? Go see a doctor. I'm an architect—why should I know what causes diarrhea anyway?"

Every person I asked acted like an authority on the subject and everybody had a different opinion about what was causing my problems. I heard everything from cancer to bacteria in my drinking water to lactose intolerance to stress to colitis. My friends and family were as ignorant about what was happening as I was, and the only thing they agreed on was that I should see a doctor, which I had no intention of doing. I would have to figure it out myself, so I began a months-long process of trial and error to see what was causing it.

I made alterations to my diet and lifestyle on a weekly basis. I wrote down everything I ate and created an "elimination diary" on my computer, listing the date, what foods I ate, and how bad my "problem" was that day. I figured that way I could look for patterns: Were certain kinds of food causing it? Were weekdays worse than weekends? Full moons? Bad weather? I made changes to my lifestyle on a daily basis, trying to identify the one thing that was causing it, or the one thing that might make it stop. I tried exercising more and tried exercising less. I cut out all dairy products from my diet, then gave up alcohol, then coffee and then spicy food. I tried sleeping with a heating pad on my stomach, and tried to get more sleep at night. I drank bottled water and ate enough bran muffins and prunes to keep a retirement community content for an entire year. I thought I was taking a pretty scientific approach to the problem, but the truth is, I didn't really know what I was doing. I never really stuck with one diet long enough to see if something was truly working or not, and when it seemed to get better for a few weeks I would revert to my normal diet and things would get bad again.

As months passed, I began to grab at straws in my attempt to cure myself. Walking into work one day I saw an audio-cassette on the ground. Thinking it might be some band I liked or something, I picked it up. I looked at the tape and read the label: "Stop Smoking Through Hypnosis." I took the tape home. I don't smoke, but I had never been hypnotized and was curious to know if it really worked. I knew that hypnosis worked for all kinds of things, but had not even considered it for my digestive troubles. I naively figured I could just listen to the tape and mentally substitute "stop having diarrhea" every time I heard "stop smoking." How different could it be? I thought.

At home that night, I told my wife that I would be downstairs and that I did not want to be disturbed for an hour or so. I listened to the tape. The man's voice on the cassette was calm and soothing and made me feel very relaxed. I sat in a large padded chair with a blanket over me, closed my eyes and listened. The hypnotist went through a number of relaxation exercises and then began to talk about losing the desire to smoke. He said I was in control of my smoking and could stop any time I wanted to. Smoking was a choice—I didn't need to smoke. He told me that when I woke up I would no longer have the desire to smoke. He gave me a hypnotic instruction that once I woke up, every time I saw the color red it would remind me how much I did not want to smoke.

Looking back, I'm sure I was never really hypnotized, but I listened intently and kept substituting "diarrhea" for "smoking," while repeating his statements in my mind. "I am in control of my diarrhea. I can stop having diarrhea any time I want to. Having diarrhea is a choice—I don't have to have diarrhea. Seeing the color red will remind me that I don't want to have diarrhea...." When I was about half way through the tape I felt a sudden sharp cramp in my gut. Bomb in the building. Heeding the warning, I got up from the chair and raced to the bathroom. I guess if you are going to do hypnosis, it probably pays to get the right kind.

For months, I tried everything I could think of to fix my problem, but nothing worked. People around me kept urging me to see a doctor, but I was adamant in my belief that I could figure it out on my own.

My cousin John had a serious drinking problem. For years he would come home from work, have five or six drinks and pass out in front of the television. His family made several attempts to get him into treatment but they were never successful. He always had excuses not to go, and in his eyes, the drinking had not messed up his life that badly so he didn't see any reason to stop. They say that alcoholics will not usually accept help until they have hit "rock bottom." They lose a job, crash the car, sleep with their best friend's mother, or something like that. When alcoholics hit "rock bottom," they realize that their situation is out of control and cannot get any worse. It is usually only then that they finally decide to get professional help.

I hit rock bottom with my digestive problems on October 17, 1998 at 2:34 in the afternoon when I went to the bathroom in my pants at work.

The day had been uneventful to that point, and I actually felt okay. I was sitting in my office preparing a budget report for the upcoming year. I was getting a lot of work done, but as I sat in my chair and innocently passed gas, I filled my pants. My eyes instantly flew wide open, and in a panic I ran out of the office. As I ran out the door, the receptionist shouted, "Hey, you forgot to sign out!" I ran with very short strides, keeping my thighs pressed together to hold the rest in.

In the men's room I was relieved to find that my dress pants had survived the incident unscathed, but my boxer shorts didn't fare as well. I did my best to clean up and ended up throwing my underwear away.

It was 20 minutes since I had run out of the office, and now I returned pale, sweating, and without my tie. The receptionist looked up from her magazine and eyed me suspiciously. "Hey. How's it going?" I said, trying to act as cool and nonchalant as possible. She rolled her eyes as I walked past. I walked into my office, closed the door, and called a gastroenterologist.

The secretary at the clinic answered, "St. Anthony's GI Specialists. Can I help you?" Nervously, I explained what had just happened to me and that I wanted to see a doctor. She told me that I could come in the following Tuesday, but that based on some of the symptoms I described, the doctor would want to do something called a sigmoidoscopy to see what was going on. I did not know what a sigmoidoscopy was but I didn't like the sound of it. I asked the secretary. Big mistake.

"A sigmoidoscopy is a procedure where the doctor examines your colon with a long flexible scope so he can see your colon and make sure there are no signs of cancer or anything like that," she said. "Okay...so, like...then he has to actually put something, you know, in me?" I asked. "Yes, the doctor has to insert a flexible scope into your rectum and move it through to your colon so that he can see what is going on," she explained. I panicked. "What?" I said, almost hyperventilating. "He has to stick a scope inside me! Are you kidding me?" She told me that no, she was not kidding and to make it worse, she added that they required that I give myself two enemas an hour before the procedure. "Two! Why two?" I asked. "I don't even know how to do an enema. Why do I have to give myself an enema at all? And why two? And how big is this scope? Is it like a microscope? And can't he diagnose me without sticking things inside me?" I must have sounded like a five-year-old getting a shot. "Sir," she said, "you have to have a sigmoidoscopy if you want to find out what is wrong with you. To do that you have to be clean inside so the doctor can see the walls of your colon. To get clean you have to give yourself two enemas. I'm sorry, but there is no way around it. It really is not that bad; most people say it doesn't hurt at all."

I get embarrassed just buying toilet paper, so the thought of buying enemas was awful. I wished you could buy them from one of those adult mail-order places where they send things in plain brown wrappers so nobody can see what you got. But since that was not an option, I went at seven in the morning to a store that was 14 miles from my home to minimize the chance of seeing someone I knew. I figured that early in the morning was the best time to go because nobody would be in the store. But when I got there I saw that the place was busy with people buying things on their way to work. Even worse was that only two checkout lanes were open, and the cashiers at both were attractive young women—definitely not the type of people I wanted to face when buying enemas. I quickly headed for the drug section of the store and found enemas stacked neatly among the laxatives and hemorrhoid creams.

Whoever designed the packaging for enemas didn't have me in mind. I hoped the box label would be subtle so that anybody who saw them in my cart might mistake them for cough syrup or saline solution, but that wasn't the case. On three sides of the box it said "ENEMA" in gigantic bold letters with a large photograph of the enema underneath. It looked like a water bottle with a straw fashioned to the top, and left little for the imagination. On the fourth panel of the box was a line drawing of a man giving himself an enema to show what position to use. The man was on his knees with his rear end stuck up in the air and his face pressed to the ground. I was sure that anyone who saw the drawing would imagine me in the same position. For a moment I considered just putting them in my coat and stealing them so that I wouldn't have to face the cute cashiers, but I knew that getting caught stealing enemas would be even more humiliating than buying them. I picked up a newspaper from the magazine aisle and rolled it around the enemas to keep them hidden.

I stood in line waiting to check out, doing my best to hide them in the newspaper. The man behind me was buying a carton of Pall Mall cigarettes. He had shoulder length curly black hair and a full beard. He was about six feet five inches tall and very well built. He was wearing a plaid flannel shirt and carpenter's overalls. He was very rugged and macho looking, and reminded me of the Marlboro Man. He was the kind of guy who intimidates the heck out of scrawny guys like me. As I stepped forward in line, one of the enemas fell out of the newspaper and landed at his feet. My face flushed red, and as I bent down to pick up the box, he snickered out loud. I thought I would die of embarrassment. When I finally got to the cashier I tried to cover by saying, "Grandma sure did pick a fine time to run out of these things." She just rolled her eyes at me.

Back home, I prepared to give myself the enemas. I closed the blinds on every window in the house, dead-bolted the doors, and locked the dog in the basement. I went into the bathroom, opened one of the enemas, and read the directions. I quickly gave myself the enemas and tried my best to relax before my appointment.

I arrived at the clinic 15 minutes early and checked in at the front desk. There were two others sitting in the waiting room—a man and a woman, both much older than I was. We all knew we were probably there for the same thing. I made eye contact with the man as I sat down, and he gave me one of those uneasy half-smiles that seems to say, "I know, man. I know." The woman glanced at me with a look that seemed more like pity than anything else.

After a few minutes a nurse came out and said, "Mr. Vogl?" I got up and the man next to me smiled again, this time as if to say, "Be strong, and Godspeed." The nurse was a nice professional woman in her 40s and put me at ease with small talk about the weather. She handed me a thin, pale blue hospital gown and told me to take off my clothes and put it on.

I sat on the cold stainless steel exam table and shivered in my gown while waiting for the doctor. Truth be told, I was scared to death. There was a knock on the door and Dr. Hughes came in and introduced himself.

He shook my hand and mumbled something about the weather being nice for this time of year, but I wasn't paying attention. I knew that in just a few minutes Dr. Hughes would be behind me giving me a sigmoidoscopy and I didn't care about the weather or anything else.

He continued the small talk in an attempt to calm me down. He said, "Well, I'm sure you are a little anxious about this procedure, but I promise it won't be that bad." I didn't believe him. In fact, I was practically crying with fear. There was a diagram of the human digestive system hanging on the wall. It showed an outline of a human torso with the digestive organs brightly colored and labeled, and it made me glad we have skin to cover everything. Dr. Hughes used his finger to trace the path that the scope would take in my digestive system. "In through the anus, through the rectum and then up and around to the very back of your colon," he said as he traced a path in the shape of a giant question mark on the diagram. Judging from the diagram, I figured it would take at least 18 feet of scope to make it all the way. Were I not in a backless hospital gown, I would have leapt from the table and ran home.

He instructed me to lie on my left side in a little ball, with my knees pulled in to my chin. He said that I might feel some slight cramping when the scope had to turn corners. He also told me that from time to time he would have to shoot air through the end of the scope to inflate the colon wall, which would give the camera a better look. He said that might hurt a little, too.

I once watched a television program about Jacques Cousteau. He had a team of divers who wanted to explore some caves deep in the Pacific Ocean. The caves were too deep for humans to dive to, so instead they sent a motorized robot called Navigator One. Navigator One was equipped with a camera and a large array of lights to see better in the dark caves. It was attached to a long tether and had big mechanical arms with clamps on front to collect anything of interest they found in the cave. While Navigator One moved slowly through the cave, a group of men and women watched from the ship on television monitors and pointed excitedly at the screen as details of the cave wall came into view. Sometimes the robot would miss a turn and bump into the wall of the cave, causing dirt and debris to scatter in front of the camera. I remember watching the program and almost cheering for Navigator One and the scientists. But all I could think of now was that poor cave—so helpless, just sitting there while a team of heartless scientists recklessly crashed a robot into its walls.

Dr. Hughes stood behind me and began the procedure. I was braced for the worst, but it never came. I kept waiting for it to really hurt, but after a few minutes, Dr. Hughes said, "Believe it or not, that's it. You can get dressed and I'll come back so we can talk about it." He left the room and I sat there half-stunned. "That was it?" I thought. "That was nothing. I can't believe I got so worked up for that."

I quickly got dressed and waited for Dr. Hughes to come back. He told me that there were no signs of cancer or any life-threatening conditions. We talked about my symptoms, my diet, my lifestyle, and all kinds of things related to my digestive problems. He told me that most likely I had a condition called irritable bowel syndrome, or IBS. He went on to explain that irritable bowel syndrome is sometimes called "spastic colon," and that millions of people have it. "Irritable bowel syndrome?" I asked, obviously annoyed. "Tell me something I don't know. Your bowels would be irritated too if you had a sigmoidoscopy. You mean to tell me that you went to medical school for seven years and all you can tell me is that I have irritable bowels? Just what the hell is irritable bowel syndrome supposed to mean, anyway?"

Dr. Hughes was patient with me and said he understood how frustrated I was. But I was angry. I had never heard of irritable bowel syndrome or IBS, and the only time I ever heard the phrase "spastic colon" was years ago when my older brother called me one. I thought irritable bowel syndrome sounded like something he just made up. I said, "Look, Doc, I'm not trying to be a jerk or anything, but basically what I hear you telling me is that irritable bowel syndrome is just a fancy name for 'I-have-no-idea-what-in-the-hell-is-causing-you-to-go-to-the-bathroom-in-your-pants-but-we-have-to-call-it-something-so-why-not-IBS,' right?" I told him that I didn't need to have a three-foot scope inserted into my rear end to tell me that my bowels were irritable; that was abundantly apparent before I came to see him. Dr. Hughes just let me rant; he'd obviously seen people react like this before.

"I can understand your frustration," he said. "but this is a very real condition that impacts millions of people. There is no cure, but there are a lot of things we can do, working together, to improve your situation." He went on to tell me that there is a lot of research going on and that every year they learn more about IBS. "There are people working on new drugs and therapies even as we speak, and one day there might even be a cure for it."

I calmed down and we talked about IBS for a long time. He told me some of the theories about what causes IBS, and what kinds of things make it worse. He gave me materials to read and made a lot of suggestions regarding diet and lifestyle. My anger and confusion started to ease, and on the drive home it hit me that at last, I finally had a name for what was wrong with me. From what Dr. Hughes told me, it would be a while before I got better, and even then I'd still have episodes. But at least I knew what I had, and I knew it was not going to kill me. On some level then, I knew I had received good news.

It is almost a year after my sigmoidoscopy, and I've pretty much accepted the fact that I have irritable bowel syndrome.

IBS is a strange condition. When people get diagnosed with things like diabetes or cancer, they usually have already heard of the conditions, and on some level, know what it means and how they should react. But even though millions of people have IBS, most people have never heard of it, and those who have usually don't want to talk about it.

One of the frustrating things about IBS is that it is isolating; millions may have it, but if nobody talks about it, you don't know. People talk about breast cancer in public forums and wear pink ribbons to show they support the cause. They made a Broadway musical about AIDS. There are public service announcements about diabetes. There are huge fund-raising walk-a-thons for kidney failure and birth defects, and support groups for epileptics. But there is little public support for IBS. Fortunately the International Foundation for Functional Gastrointestinal Disorders is beginning to create public awareness of IBS.

I used to wonder what it would be like if IBS was a condition that was more out in the open. What if actors at the Academy Awards wore brown ribbons to show support for IBS? What if they wrote a musical about a group of young people with chronic diarrhea who have to run off the stage in the middle of songs, holding their guts because they have to find a bathroom? And what if they had a walk-a-thon for IBS called "Walk for

Diarrhea"? But I know those things are never going to happen. People don't want to talk about their bowel movements in public, and I've pretty much accepted the fact that IBS can be isolating.

I still am afraid to drive across Utah because the rest stops are too infrequent. I still occasionally have to run out of the room in the middle of a conversation to get to a bathroom. I'm 30 years old and I now keep a change of underwear in my office, my briefcase, and my car just in case. And I still have bad dreams about my sigmoidoscopy and have panic attacks if I have to drive through a tunnel. I know what foods to avoid and I watch my stress and exercise regularly. My symptoms have not disappeared, but they have improved a great deal. Much of the time, I'm fine and never think about my IBS. But that usually leads to trouble because I get complacent about prevention.

One Saturday night I was at the movies with my wife. It was one of those action-suspense flicks with a lot of explosions and chase scenes. About an hour and a half into the movie the action really started to pick up when the hero got captured by the bad guys. The suspense was strong and everybody in the theater was wondering how he was going to get out of the situation—everybody but me, that is. I had forgotten to take my fiber for a few days. At dinner before the movie I ate food on my "danger list." I suddenly felt the all-too-familiar "Brrrrup. Brooop. Grrrr-ooop" of gas rumbling in my abdomen, and all I cared about was finding the rest room. I excused myself and climbed over my wife to get to the aisle. "Again?" she whispered. I didn't answer. The message my body was sending me was a familiar one: forget the movie and get to a bathroom—now!

Your body talks to you. My body screams at me.

"There is a bomb in the building. You have two minutes." Click. Dial tone.

CHAPTER 1

Facing the Facts

IRRITABLE BOWEL SYNDROME, spastic colon, spastic colitis, mucous colitis, nervous stomach, nervous diarrhea, functional bowel disease—the names may vary, but one fact is certain: suffering from this symptomatic disorder is no fun. It can cause embarrassment, create suspicion, harm relationships, shorten vacation trips, spoil parties, and turn gregarious people into recluses. The medical term most frequently used today is irritable bowel syndrome, or IBS, and there are still others that may represent variants of IBS, namely esophageal spasm, aerophagia, nonulcer dyspepsia, and proctalgia fugax.

IBS is the most common of all gastrointestinal (GI) disorders, affecting as many as one in five adults in North America, or 20 percent of the population in the United States. IBS significantly decreases the quality of life of those who suffer from it. It is estimated that IBS sufferers miss three times as many days from work and school compared to those without the disorder. And yet, only an estimated 25 percent of those with IBS seek medical help.

This perplexing problem is the leading cause of chronic, recurrent abdominal pain, referred to as "gas pains" by some sufferers. The discomfort is linked with embarrassing symptoms such as sudden, unexpected bouts of diarrhea, belching, and excessive gas. Intermittent or chronic constipation is also common. People with uncontrolled IBS are rarely "regular"; their bowel movements tend to be either too fast or too slow.

I am not certain the term "irritable bowel syndrome" is the most descriptive or even the most accurate. Perhaps "sensitive bowel syndrome" would be more in line with the symptoms and feelings of sufferers. "Irritable bowel syndrome" has negative connotations that make sufferers feel that they, somehow, are personally responsible for their condition. Indeed more recent literature has shown that IBS sufferers have "hypersensitive" responses to various stimuli in the gut resulting in the pain, bloating, and bowel dysfunction experienced.

The fact is, the majority of the population can eat and drink as it pleases, without suffering intense cramps and altered patterns of bowel movements. Those with IBS have guts that are "sensitive" to various edibles (triggers) that the average person tolerates without difficulty. However, marked improvement is possible.

Profile of an IBS Sufferer

In my experience treating those suffering from IBS, I can say that there is no exclusive profile of a person with this disorder. Single, married, student, professional, craftsperson, homemaker—all can be affected. Some are unaware that they suffer from IBS; others have come to believe their abnormal bowel function is without remedy, and thus no longer seek qualified medical treatment.

I have listened with a sympathetic

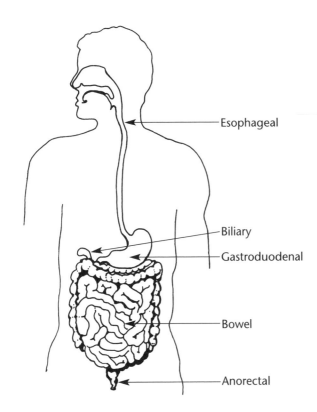

Esophageal

Biliary

Gastroduodenal

Bowel

Anorectal

IBS is one of over 20 functional GI disorders, but the most common one in North America. The functional GI disorders are separated into five regions of the gastrointestinal tract, as illustrated.

ear to countless stories such as the one told by Matt Vogl of the annoyance, pain, and embarrassment caused by IBS symptoms. I have heard stories of shopping carts left unattended, of boardrooms awaiting the return of the presenter, of times of dire need when there was no change for the pay toilet. Then there was the desirable new date suddenly and mysteriously left alone several times during dinner, wondering what he may have done wrong. I recall the story of the college freshman who bolted from the classroom on several occasions during an exam "to relieve myself," leading the instructor to suspect that the student was hiding cheat sheets in the rest room.

Facts about Women and IBS

- 20 percent of the North American population suffers from IBS, and 70 percent of these sufferers are women.
- Fibromyalgia syndrome (FMS) shares many common features with IBS and occurs more frequently in women than in men.
- Up to 50 percent of women with more severe IBS seen by GI specialists have a past history of sexual or physical abuse in childhood.

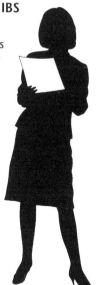

Having IBS or spastic colon may mean going to an unfamiliar establishment and immediately having to locate the rest room in case you get an urgent call. It may mean acquainting yourself with all the rest stops along the route before you take an automobile trip. Female sufferers describe the anxiety of coping with long lines and jammed rest rooms at public events. "I won't go to a football game with my husband, because the fear of making it to the john is enough to trigger symptoms," one woman told me. The availability and accessibility of rest rooms becomes a major life issue.

IBS is symptomatic. That is, we recognize the disorder in a set of symptoms. Not all sufferers experience identical symptoms, a factor that clouds instant diagnosis. The theory is, treat the symptoms, and the disorder will often lapse into remission. And practice generally confirms this theory.

IBS is not new, but I truly believe it is becoming more prevalent. Our hurry-up lifestyles emphasizing early achievement and super-success clearly foster unbearable stresses, poor eating habits, and little time to nurture one's self-esteem. For those who are predisposed to develop IBS, modern lifestyles create the "perfect" environment to cultivate this disorder.

For example, Theresa was the last person anyone would expect to see in a doctor's office. She was young and, on the surface, appeared very healthy. A member of a local health club, she worked out regularly, was in good physical condition, and was very diet conscious. On her first visit to me, she complained of a "burning pain" in the pit of her stomach, and bowel movements that were either too loose or too hard. "I never seem to have a regular bowel movement," she said.

These symptoms first appeared, I discovered, shortly after a promotion at work and usually occurred during times of stress, particularly while Theresa was at work. I first obtained an X ray of the upper gastrointestinal tract to rule out an ulcer and made a tentative diagnosis of IBS. We also discussed Theresa's lack of self-confidence, particularly in her new position at work. After she had explored this idea, she was able to help herself through simple assertiveness training.

Today Theresa's symptoms are well under control as a result of a changed attitude about herself. She is on her way to achieving an enhanced state of mental, physical, and social well-being. For Theresa, treating the symptoms had a great deal to do with the way she perceived herself and her worth.

While IBS is equally prevalent around the world, it occurs twice as frequently in women as in men in North America. In India and Sri Lanka, however, estimates show a higher incidence of IBS in males than females. One possible explanation for these gender differences is that cultural factors determine who seeks medical care, and these cultural factors are more important than gender.

At this point, you may be wondering why, if IBS is so common, you haven't heard more about it. The fact is that the topic of our bowel functions arises only infrequently during everyday conversation. It is as if this subject is too personal, making its discussion taboo.

Increased Support and Research

Fortunately, IBS has been receiving long-overdue attention. Until recently, scientific understanding of IBS has been very limited. IBS has no structural or "organic cause," and consequently the disorder is classified as "functional" and the symptoms treated. Over the last two decades, there has been a significant increase in medical research about all the functional gastrointestinal disorders, resulting in improved diagnosis and treatment of IBS. In 1988, the first Rome criteria for diagnosing IBS were presented at the 13th International Congress of Gastroenterology. A decade later the criteria were refined and expanded to include all the functional GI disorders. In 1999 the Rome II criteria were published, and are discussed in the next chapter.

The pharmaceutical industry has also increased its research of treatment for IBS in recent years. A new class of medications are being investigated, based on research into the connection between the central and enteric nervous systems. It is a promising sign that IBS is finally being taken seriously as a legitimate disorder by the spectrum of scientific investigators.

In 1995, the First International Symposium on Functional Gastrointestinal Disorders convened in Milwaukee, Wisconsin, sponsored by the International Foundation for Functional Gastrointestinal Disorders (IFFGD). Since then, international symposiums have occurred every two years. The IFFGD also conducts public awareness campaigns, produces educational materials, and lobbies for continued research and support by industry and government.

While there is, as yet, no final cure for IBS, increased research and growing public support are improving diagnosis and treatment. I have found that many people respond favorably to a combination of treatments discussed in the following chapters. Today, those suffering from IBS are able to take part in normal daily activities, which previously would have been often impossible to attain.

CHAPTER 2

Diagnosing IBS
and Getting Help

IRRITABLE BOWEL SYNDROME has had several names in the past, the most common of which is spastic colon. Other terms have included "spastic colitis," "mucous colitis," and "nervous stomach." Since "colitis" implies inflammation of the colon—and since IBS involves no inflammation and is not limited to the colon—this term is generally no longer used. "Irritable" bowel syndrome, in contrast, implies an irritability of the entire bowel. A syndrome is a group of symptoms or signs that occur together and produce a pattern typical of a particular disorder. Thus, irritable bowel syndrome is a group of symptoms involving the entire digestive tract, the alimentary canal.

Irritable bowel syndrome was first described in North America in 1817, and appeared in the English medical literature over the following years. Some early accounts emphasized passage of "membranes" in the stool, perhaps because only the most severe examples were recognized, and because most cases reported involved the abuse of purgatives or enemas. In the mid-19th century, a physician reported with amazement that the bowels could be constipated and lax in the same person. Over a century of medical misunderstanding followed, which included dismissing IBS as purely psychosomatic.

By the 1950s, physicians thought that abnormal gut motility was the basis of IBS symptoms because studies showed the condition was present in patients with abdominal pain and altered bowel function. But later studies concluded that abnormal gut motility also occurs in response to stress among those without IBS or with other disorders.

Then in 1978, Dr. Manning and colleagues published "Towards Positive Diagnosis of the Irritable Bowel" in the *British Medical Journal*. They described their efforts to identify a set of symptoms that could be used for diagnosing IBS. A decade later, the Manning criteria pointed out six common symptoms of IBS—abdominal pain in combination with two or more of the following features: abdominal swelling, pain relief with bowel movement, more frequent stools with onset of pain, looser stools with onset of pain, mucus in the stool, and/or a sensation of incomplete evacuation.

Rome II Diagnostic Criteria for IBS

At least 12 weeks in the previous 12 months of continuous or recurrent abdominal discomfort or pain that has two of the following three features:
• relieved with defecation
• onset is associated with a change in the frequency of stool
• onset is associated with a change in the form of stool

The Manning criteria were used successfully in many studies to define IBS for further scientific investigation. Then in the 1980s, a group of international investigators interested in functional bowel disorders met in Rome, Italy and established the Rome criteria. Although the Manning and Rome criteria gained wide acceptance among researchers, physicians were not using them in diagnosing their patients. In an effort to make the criteria more "user-friendly," the Rome II criteria were developed and published in 1999.

The Rome II criteria represent a conceptual shift in the understanding and diagnosis of functional gastrointestinal disorders. Since the 1700s, Western medicine has looked for a structural or biochemical cause to diagnose and treat illness. It is likely due to this disease-based, reductionist model that IBS has puzzled both physicians and patients alike.

Today the medical community is beginning to recognize the connection between the mind and the body, which is referred to as the biopsychosocial model. This model is enabling researchers to find connections between the brain and gut, or the central and enteric nervous systems, which is shedding light on possible causes of and medications for IBS (see Chapters 3 and 14). The biopyschosocial model is also allowing us to consider treatment options such as relaxation training and biofeed-back (see Chapter 9).

Symptoms of IBS

The Rome II criteria simply state that the cardinal feature of IBS is abdominal pain, and the pain is associated with altered bowel movement. If you don't have abdominal pain, then technically speaking, you don't have IBS. Instead, you may have functional diarrhea or functional constipation. Abdominal pain is the most frequent complaint of IBS sufferers, and the pain patterns are quite diverse. Different sufferers describe it as aching, cramping, burning, or sharp. The pains can be relatively constant but are more commonly intermittent.

The defecation pattern of IBS may consist of constipation, or diarrhea, or a pattern of constipation alternating with diarrhea. The more common IBS sufferer experiences abdominal cramps and urgency followed by loose bowel movements. A smaller percentage of those with IBS have harder stools that are difficult to pass with the onset of abdominal pain. A rarer condition among adults is abdominal cramps with little altered bowel function. However, children and adolescents with IBS often complain of abdominal pain only. (See Chapter 13, "GI Disorders in Children and Adolescents.")

The urge to have a bowel movement is often sudden and is experienced along with a cramping pain that is relieved after the passage of feces or gas. After the bowel movement, there may be a sense of incomplete evacuation, as if there were a fullness in the rectum, suggesting evacuation is not finished.

Often people complain of belching, bloating, nausea, decreased appetite, and excessive gas. Researchers have described other characteristics that may not involve the gut but are found more frequently in IBS sufferers than in the normal population. These include frequency of urination, incomplete emptying of the bladder, an unpleasant taste in the mouth, fatigue, and uncomfortable intercourse in women.

Some people may have multiple medical complaints, including bowel complaints, and they may be more inclined to discuss those aches, pains, and concerns that they find less embarrassing. For example, IBS seems to occur more commonly in stress-prone individuals, and they often exhibit other manifestations of stress, including tension headaches, dizziness, fatigue, diffuse muscular aches, palpitations, chest pain, and tingling of the hands and feet.

Most IBS sufferers experience mild to moderate symptoms, with about five to ten percent having severe symptoms. An estimated 75 percent of those suffering from IBS in North America do not report their complaint to a physician. However, the disorder is the most common gastrointestinal diagnosis among gastroenterologists in the U.S. If you suspect that you have the IBS symptoms described above, refer to the questionnaire in Appendix 1, "Do You Have IBS? A Checklist for You."

IBS symptoms commonly coexist with various other disorders. For example, you may experience them in conjunction with premenstrual syndrome (PMS) or with fibromyalgia syndrome (FMS). FMS is a disorder of unknown cause, characterized by generalized aching and stiffness. The major symptoms of these two disorders may predominate and prompt you to consult your physician. You should take care to discuss the disordered bowel function in addition to the other symptoms, which may overshadow the intestinal complaint. (See Chapter 16, "Facts about Coexisting Conditions," for a complete discussion of PMS and FMS.)

The Diagnostic and Treatment Steps

The greatest success in treating IBS symptoms comes from following an established approach to diagnosis and treatment of any disease: establishing the diagnosis; searching for aggravating factors; recommending appropriate lifestyle changes; judiciously using medications, if needed; and projecting an expected outcome.

The approach to diagnosing IBS varies with a person's age, duration of his or her symptoms, and the most prevalent symptoms experienced. The first step, establishing the diagnosis, is probably the most important one. For some people, a diagnosis can be difficult to make, as symptoms may differ from those of the classic case. They may present a confusing picture to the physician, who then may believe that extensive testing is warranted. Others may come with symptoms described by the Rome II criteria and obvious triggers, which when avoided, lead to prompt resolution of symptoms. When this happens, exhaustive testing may not be necessary. Thus, the length of time it takes to establish a diagnosis of IBS and to find effective treatment often varies a great deal.

Unfortunately, many people have come to me only after attempting to treat themselves with over-the-counter remedies for their diarrhea, constipation, or abdominal pain, before being systematically evaluated for the cause of these symptoms. Before treating these symptoms, it is most important to discover their cause.

The second step is to check for aggravating factors. For instance, I have found that many people with IBS symptoms have a coexisting dairy product (lactose) intolerance. Avoiding dairy products or using lactase enzyme supplements has often led to resolution or a marked improvement of symptoms in this group. In addition, hidden food sensitivities, improper exercise, other poor lifestyle habits, and stress can each aggravate digestive problems.

The third step is to make significant changes in lifestyle. This step is calculated to help individuals become as healthy as they can possibly be and involves five basic areas: proper diet; exercise; stress reduction; moderation in daily living; and finding a social sense of well-being. The World Health Organization (WHO) has defined health as the complete stage of mental, physical, and social well-being. Although I have not encountered anyone who has been able to totally achieve this stage, it is certainly a worthwhile goal.

Lack of exercise, stress, and poor dietary habits can have direct effects on the digestive tract. These factors may also lead to such problems as hypertension, diabetes, and obesity. In turn, such disorders and the medications taken to treat them may adversely affect the gut. So by taking steps to ensure your general health, you will be better able to ensure your digestive health as well.

To have a social sense of well-being means to feel comfortable in social situations. Finding a social sense of well-being is important, because it helps to enhance the self-esteem necessary to prevent depression and anxiety. You should feel good about who you are and why you are here; this attitude will give you a positive sense of control over your life and prevent mood disorders, which may lead to overeating or lack of appetite.

You may not necessarily need attention in all five areas, but if you want to be as healthy as possible, analyze your personal situation to determine the areas in which you may need to improve. Some changes may be as simple as 20 minutes of exercise three times a week and watching your intake of certain food groups. Other changes may be more complicated, and take more time, and what works for you may not work for someone else.

The fourth step—the judicious use of medications—is employed only after aggravating factors have been eliminated and appropriate lifestyle changes made, without the complete removal of symptoms.

The final step is to project an expected outcome. Whereas a percentage of IBS sufferers experience spontaneous remission and become virtually symptom free, for the majority, recurring symptoms will remain a concern. The primary goal is to help you live successfully with this disorder, minimizing symptoms as much as possible. It is important to realize this so that you will not become discouraged if symptoms recur after a long symptom-free interval.

Testing

Physicians may vary somewhat in their approach to problem solving. As explained earlier, there is no single conclusive test available to diagnose IBS. I begin the diagnosis with what I consider the most important first step: a detailed clinical history followed by a physical exam. I look for the IBS symptoms and the absence of so-called red flags. The red flags are symptoms or conditions which suggest the existence of an alternative or coexisting disease; these are fever, weight loss, anemia, persistent diarrhea, severe constipation, rectal bleeding, night-time symptoms of pain and abnormal bowel function, new onset of symptoms in those 50 years of age and older (IBS usually begins earlier in life), and a family history of

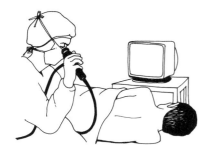

Diagnostic Tests

- Blood tests
- X-rays
- Endoscopy:
  Sigmoidoscopy,
  Colonoscopy

Reproduced with permission from the International
Foundation for Functional Gastrointestinal Disorders.

digestive tract cancer, inflamma-tory bowel disease, or celiac disease.

Next, I order a limited number of routine screening tests, such as blood tests, a urinalysis, and a stool specimen test to check for blood in the stool or for bowel infection. There may be other, more special-ized tests, to exclude the presence of any diseases or pathological disor-ders suggested by the history and exam. These procedures are followed to exclude other diseases or disorders that may produce similar symp-toms. For example, I ordered an upper gastrointestinal X ray for Theresa's case (discussed in Chapter 1) to rule out an ulcer as the cause of the burning pain she reported.

For others, more thorough testing may be necessary. Charles, a 55-year-old college professor, complained of worsening constipation and sharp abdominal pains. His medical history revealed a lot of "colic" while he was growing up, although he had been free of symptoms for many years. Because of his age and symptoms, I ordered a colonoscopy (the visual examination of the lining of the large intestine using a fiber-optic instrument) to exclude the possibility of colon cancer. When these tests returned normal, I recommended a gradual increase in dietary fiber. Charles has since done quite well.

Others, by the nature of the discomforts, may warrant gallbladder tests or direct visual inspection of the digestive tract by endoscopy. When all tests prove inconclusive, or when I see a patient who I believe is suffering from IBS but who is not responding to treatment, I may refer him or her to a gastroenterologist for a second opinion. As an internist, I often consult with other specialists in their respective disciplines.

Gastroenterologists are physicians who specialize in the treatment of digestive disorders. I will refer a patient for a second opinion if I am un-sure of the diagnosis, or if there is or has been unsatisfactory response to treatment. Conversely, if I am confident of the diagnosis and the patient is feeling well, referral is not necessary. In addition, gastroenterologists are trained to do the specialized tests that may be required when a diagnosis of IBS is not clear. If possible try to find a primary care physician or gastroenterologist with a special interest in functional bowel disorders.

Choosing a Doctor

You may or may not be under the care of a physician for your bowel complaints. If not, I encourage you to find one. Whom should you see? How do you choose a doctor? These are important questions that need to be addressed.

The best time to choose a doctor is before you urgently need one. Choosing a doctor before an emergency occurs allows you the opportunity to do some research into the doctor's qualifications and references, the nature of the practice, office hours, hospital affiliations, and so on. Ask those you trust to suggest a physician, or ask if they know anything about a doctor you are considering. Many local hospitals and medical societies have physician-referral services. See if you can set up a brief "get-acquainted" visit with the doctor you have chosen. (The initial charge, if any, will be well spent in the long run.)

Signs and symptoms not usually associated with IBS:

- blood in the stool
- fever
- weight loss
- onset at 50 years of age or more
- night-time symptoms
- family history of GI cancer, inflammatory bowel disease or celiac disease
- recent onset of symptoms, especially in those 40 years of age or more
- abnormal laboratory test results

Another question is whether you should see a specialist. I suggest you first see a primary-care physician (family practitioner, internist, or pediatrician). Odds are that he or she will be able to suggest an effective evaluation and treatment plan. If you are not given a treatment plan to address your symptoms, ask your primary-care physician to recommend a gastroenterologist. Many specialists prefer—or may even require—that you have an established primary-care physician. The primary-care physician is in a better position to treat the whole patient, focusing not only on the digestive system but on the interrelationship of all body systems as well. If you are a woman, you may have an established relationship with an obstetrician/gynecologist, with whom you can discuss your digestive disorder to obtain recommendations regarding evaluation, treatment, or referral.

During the first visit to your doctor, he or she will gather useful information about your digestive problem. The most important step in establishing a diagnosis of IBS is to obtain a detailed clinical history. Many medical authorities now contend that a correct diagnosis can be made on the basis of the Rome II criteria, the absence of "red flags," and normal initial screening tests. This is fortunate, since it makes extensive testing unnecessary. This is not to say that certain tests may not be required to rule out other disorders. Common tests used to evaluate the gastrointestinal tract are discussed in Chapter 18, "Common Tests You May Face," and Chapter 17, "Other Common Gastrointestinal Disorders," describes other common gastrointestinal conditions.

CHAPTER 3

Causes, Triggers, and Risk Factors

I ONCE ATTENDED a medical lecture on high blood pressure. After the lecture, a physician in the audience posed a very thought-provoking question to the guest speaker, a visitor from a prestigious medical university. The speaker paused briefly, then replied, "That is a very good question. If I were a medical student, I would answer, 'I don't know.' As a professor of medicine, I must state, 'The answer is not known.'" It is the same for the question "What causes irritable bowel syndrome?" The answer is not known. We understand what happens; we just don't have a complete understanding of why it happens.

Disordered Rhythm in the Gastrointestinal Tract

Although the exact cause of IBS is unknown, and it is unlikely that there is a single cause for the disorder, the common denominator among sufferers seems to be a disordered rhythm in the gastrointestinal tract. As described in "Your Internal Food Processor" on pages 32–33, normal movement of intestinal contents depends on the orderly contractile rhythm of the intestinal smooth muscle—the movement known as peristalsis. When this natural rhythm of bowel muscle is disrupted, problems arise.

Intestinal contractions consist of "segmental contractions" (which essentially mix and churn intestinal contents), and "propulsive contrac-

Your Internal Food Processor

Digestion works like a giant food processor, using both mechanical and chemical means to break down the food you eat into elements suitable for your body to use. Our digestive system consists of the alimentary canal and its glands. In its most basic sense, the alimentary canal is a hollow tube some 27 feet long. In the 15 to 72 hours it takes a meal to pass through, the alimentary canal adds chemicals and hormones, mixes well, extracts nutrients and water, and reserves the refuse for elimination.

The Role of the Brain

Your brain is the first organ involved in digestion, and just the thought, sight, or smell of food is enough for it to initiate the secretion of digestive juices and saliva. The next time you anticipate a well-prepared meal or holiday feast, notice if you begin to salivate. By the time you sit down at the table, your "food processor" will be primed and ready to go.

Chewing

As soon as you take a bite of food, you begin the second phase of digestion: chewing. Chewing has several functions: it tears the food into smaller pieces for easier swallowing, exposes a greater surface to digestive fluids, and mixes it with saliva and mucin. Chewing and swallowing, incidentally, are the only conscious acts of digestion. After that, the autonomic nervous system takes over and you're on automatic pilot.

Dentists have observed that the oral cavity must be in optimal operating order to ensure proper function. Periodontal disease, developmental abnormalities, poorly fitting dentures, or mechanical injury of your teeth, jaw, and supporting structures can lead to inadequate or painful chewing. If your ability to chew food is impaired, consider a dental evaluation and take any necessary steps to correct problems.

Swallowing

When you swallow, your esophagus—the portion of the alimentary canal between your mouth and stomach—propels each bolus, or portion of food, to your waiting stomach. The act of swallowing involves an action known as peristalsis, in which the muscles of your esophagus establish a wavelike rhythm of contractions that propel the bolus along its way, much like squeezing a toothpaste tube causes toothpaste to move through the tube and eventually squirt out. This action is so efficient that you can swallow even when you are upside down. Some of the problems encountered with IBS stem from an interruption in the normal timing and rhythmical action of peristalsis.

Moving Food through the Stomach and Intestines

The stomach, which is the widest portion of the alimentary canal, serves as a sort of waiting room and preparation chamber. The stomach releases acids to assist in breaking down food particles; it also releases mucus to protect the stomach lining from acid burns. The stomach continues a rhythmical movement to mix the food with stomach acid, turning the food into a semi-digested material called chyme.

Through peristaltic movement, successive amounts of chyme enter the first part of the small intestine, called the duodenum. The small intestine is so named because of its diameter. It is actually some 21 feet long and extends from the stomach to the large intestine.

In the duodenum, chyme comes into contact with enzymes from the pancreas and bile from the gallbladder. The pancreas produces the enzymes protease, amylase, and lipase. These assist, respectively, in breaking down proteins into amino acids, complex carbohydrates into simple sugars, and fat into fatty acids.

Bile is manufactured in the liver and stored in the gallbladder. It acts as an emulsifier by dividing fats into smaller particles that will become suspended in water. This allows fats—which do not mix well with water—to be more easily absorbed, in the same way that detergents break up grease. Bile acids are a constituent of bile and may be irritating to the intestines. In some people, excessive bile acids may enter the intestinal tract, causing diarrhea. This excess bile acid secretion is one of the newer theories that might explain IBS symptoms in susceptible individuals. It is fairly common in patients who have recently had a cholecystectomy (surgical removal of the gallbladder).

The small intestine contains many folds and fingerlike projections called "villi." Villi absorb the component parts of chyme—amino acids, simple sugars, and fatty acids—and pass them through the bloodstream into the liver for additional modification and use throughout your body. Damage to small intestinal villi can occur as a result of wheat or gluten sensitivity producing a malabsorptive syndrome which may mimic irritable bowel syndrome.

Indigestible parts of your food move from the small intestine into the large intestine. The large intestine, or colon, is approximately three feet long and consists of the cecum, ascending colon, transverse colon, descending colon, sigmoid, and rectum. Although these names refer to different segments of the large intestine, it functions as a unit, absorbing excess water and storing digestive by-products until elimination.

The normal rhythm of peristalsis moves food along the entire digestive system. When this normal action is interrupted by such factors as diet or emotional stress, the result is often the discomfort experienced by those suffering from IBS.

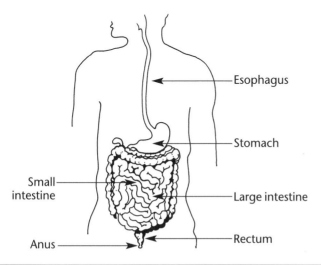

Normal Function of the Bowels

Food partly digested in stomach
▼
Moves through small intestine; digested
▼
Feces enter large intestine
▼
Move to rectum
▼
Eliminated through anus

Reproduced with permission from the International Foundation for Functional Gastrointestinal Disorders.

tions" (which move intestinal contents forward). During periods of exaggerated segmental contractions, someone may experience abdominal cramps, bloating, and constipation. Forward movement decreases, and the stools become hard and compressed, making them difficult to pass.

Imagine, for a moment, that you are holding in both hands a long, thin balloon and that this balloon represents a portion of your intestinal tract. Suddenly, you squeeze with both hands and the center of the balloon bulges. This is similar to what happens when segmented contractions are amplified, which produces painful cramps or spasms.

Exaggerated propulsive contractions lead to bowel movements that are loose and frequent. People with this condition may also feel a sense of urgency, experiencing a sudden need for a bowel movement as they frantically search for the nearest rest room.

In some ways, IBS is analogous to asthma. In fact, IBS has been referred to as "asthma of the bowel." Like the hollow intestinal tract, the hollow bronchial breathing tubes contain sheets of smooth muscle fibers. Various stimuli, including emotional stress, inhaled irritants, and food substances, can trigger contractions of bronchial smooth muscle, resulting in breathlessness and wheezing.

Additionally, irritable bowel syndrome may be considered analogous to migraine headaches. This disorder has a hereditary predisposition. These headaches begin with the contraction of smooth muscles in blood vessels of the brain. This is followed by dilation of these same blood vessels, resulting in a "pounding" headache. Stress as well as various dietary triggers (MSG, red wine, etc.) are responsible for development of migraine headaches.

Heightened Sensitivity of the Gut

Just as disordered rhythm of the intestines is a condition of IBS, so too is increased sensitivity of the gut a common, though not universal, symptom. Current studies on the connections between the central nervous system (CNS) and the nervous system of the gastrointestinal tract (called the enteric nervous system—ENS) are finding more pieces of the IBS puzzle. For example, it appears that the CNS plays a role in IBS because IBS symptoms usually cease with sleep.

The nervous system is made up of the brain and spinal cord (the CNS) and the peripheral nervous system, comprised of motor and sensory nerves. The CNS controls consciousness and voluntary actions. Part of the peripheral nervous system is the autonomic nervous system, which regulates involuntary functions of the body such as your heart beat. The autonomic system also controls the ENS, which is responsible for smooth muscle contraction, blood flow, and movement of fluids and electrolytes in the gut.

Some researchers think that abnormalities in the CNS and ENS regulation of the bowel among those with IBS may result from inherent differences in individuals and their nervous systems. This may explain why IBS symptoms vary so much among individuals. Researchers are also finding that IBS sufferers have decreased thresholds for pain. In a study in which a rectal balloon was inserted in the rectum of individuals with and without IBS, both painful and nonpainful sensations were experienced by IBS sufferers at significantly low balloon volumes. Some also experienced pain in the back, shoulders, thighs, and chest during this study, which points to a problem in the central processing of visceral sensations among IBS sufferers.

Recent research into the "brain-gut" connection has increased understanding of the various neurotransmitters responsible for the functioning of the ENS. (A neurotransmitter is a chemical involved in the sending of nerve signals between nerves.) The neurotransmitter serotonin is a major player in the motility of the gastrointestinal tract. It is believed that release of serotonin from the lining of the gut starts the peristalic process of digestion. There are various medications currently being studied that affect the nerve receivers of serotonin in an attempt to control IBS symptoms.

Brain-Gut Connection

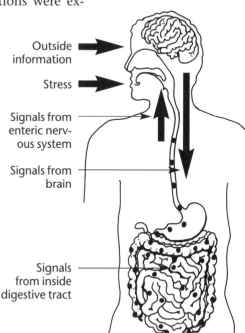

Outside information

Stress

Signals from enteric nervous system

Signals from brain

Signals from inside digestive tract

The Theory of Multiple Causes

When physicians consider the causes of any functional disorder or organic disease, they consider all the factors that may be involved—the cause, the condition of the patient, and the way the body is affected. While single causes of IBS have been suggested—such as lack of dietary fiber, abnormal responses of the gastrointestinal tract to emotional stress, abnormal central processing of visceral sensations, and specific food intolerance or sensitivities—as it turns out, all may be causes to varying degrees in different people. In fact, some authorities have divided patients into subgroups called "food reactors," "psychological reactors," and "mixed reactors." One authority states that "irritable bowel syndrome is not likely to be a single disorder, but rather a spectrum of disorders resulting from disturbances at all levels of the gut."

A study that supports the theory of multiple causes categorized IBS patients into chronic and recent-onset (within the past two years). Both groups had symptoms that were similar in severity, although those with chronic IBS had significantly more psychological symptoms. Over an 18-month period of treatment, those with chronic IBS had little or no improvement of symptoms, while those with recent-onset improved significantly, especially with regard to abdominal pain.

People with chronic IBS often have psychological symptoms (in particular, anxiety and depression) at the same time, and may experience more severe pain than those with recent-onset IBS. Chronic IBS often begins in childhood or adolescence. In one study, almost half of those with recurrent abdominal pain in childhood had symptoms of IBS 30 years later. Researchers have suggested that symptoms of IBS may develop as the result of "learned illness behavior"; adults who now have IBS were given special consideration and "treats" when they experienced abdominal pain as children.

Triggers

The digestive system of every individual functions differently as well, and there are various factors that may trigger symptoms in any given individual. These factors include the timing and content of meals, stressful situations, and various hormones. For example, eating a meal that is high in fat (like fried chicken) stimulates the release of a hormone called cholecystokinin. Cholecystokinin is, among other things, a potent stimulus for propulsive contractions of the colon. In some cases, I believe that this may account for worsening symptoms immediately after ingestion of a fatty meal. Other dietary triggers are gas-producing foods, lactose, sorbitol, fructose, and caffeine.

The use of antibiotics, which reduces the microorganisms (called "flora") normally occurring in the bowel, may be another trigger for IBS. Alternatively, a study published in the December 2000 issue of the *American Journal of Gastroenterology* suggests a percentage of IBS patients had overgrowth of bacteria in the small intestine and benefitted from antibiotic treatment. Understanding the balance between "good" and "bad" bacteria in the gut may hold some answers and improve our current understanding of IBS. Although results are not conclusive, several studies showed that patients with IBS improved when they received natural intestinal flora.

About one-third of people with IBS say that their symptoms begin after having gastroenteritis or other intestinal infections. In the case of gastroenteritis, IBS symptoms may be triggered by the imbalance of digestive enzymes in the intestinal lining resulting from the infection, creating a temporary lactose intolerance for example. Alternately, the stimulation of nerve fibers that mediate pain during the infection become chronically stimulated—like a burglar alarm that won't shut off.

Surgery may also be a trigger for IBS. Damage to nerve endings may increase the perception of gastrointestinal symptoms by stimulating nerves from the gut that lead to the brain.

Stress itself may exacerbate IBS symptoms by disturbing the intestine's motility. Common examples are the "butterflies in the stomach" or "nervous diarrhea" that most people have at some time experienced before moments of high stress. Numerous studies show that increased activity of the colon, stomach, and small intestine occur during stress, anger, and aggressive reactions. In one study, a person was informed during an examination of the rectum and lower colon that cancer had been found, and the news caused immediate contractions of the lower colon. Upon hearing the news that this was a hoax—that there was in fact no cancer—the contractions stopped. For a detailed discussion of how stress can affect the intestinal tract, see Chapter 9.

Risk Factors

There are no confirmed risk factors for IBS aside from being alive, but ongoing research reveals several possibilities. While IBS affects people of all ages, it may begin early in life, peak during middle age, and decline after the age of 65. IBS appears to run in the family; children of parents with IBS are more likely to report IBS symptoms than other children; a genetic tendency may be involved, but family behavior patterns may be more influential.

Researchers are investigating the possibility that the intestinal tract might be sensitized by trauma, inflammation, and infection. One study has found that the risk of developing IBS is ten times higher in those with recent bacterial gastroenteritis. Other research indicates that many IBS sufferers were victims of physical or sexual abuse earlier in life. Abuse may alter CNS processing of painful sensations, thereby increasing the experience of pain and altering a person's ability to cope with it. Victims of abuse tend to have more severe cases of IBS and one study indicates that they also tend to have poor health overall.

My own observations suggest that it is difficult to determine whether and how much psychological and physical factors contribute to the development of IBS symptoms. The key is to realize that both psychological factors and physical factors must be investigated in tracking down causes of IBS. It is not a question of whether or not symptoms have a psychological origin versus a physical cause; rather the compelling question is which part each factor plays in the development of symptoms.

The following chapters cover the effects of proper diet, fiber, and food sensitivities, and how to effectively deal with emotional stress. If you have IBS, you are the specialist for your particular symptoms. However, you should see your physician, because he or she is the specialist who can determine which mechanisms may underlie your symptoms. Only by working together will you be able to discover what is causing irritable bowel syndrome in your particular case.

CHAPTER 4

What You Should Know About Diet

WE ALL NEED proper nutrition for our general good health, but proper nutrition is absolutely essential for those with chronic digestive disorders such as IBS. Your body responds automatically when you eat. In fact, it must react to the meal to set in motion the normal digestive process, which allows your body to extract the nutrients it needs. Eating, for most, is one of life's greater pleasures. However, for those suffering from IBS, it can be a painful, annoying experience. This chapter presents general dietary recommendations that hopefully will help you understand how certain foods may cause pain and other unpleasant symptoms.

Recipe for Indigestion

Warren is an important publishing executive. His days are filled with deadlines, and there are never enough hours in a day to meet them all. He rushes out to lunch, taking a sheaf of contracts with him, and orders hastily from a menu in a crowded café. He drinks coffee while he waits. "If I could only dispense with the time it takes to eat," he thinks, "I would have time to review the Thompson proposal before that meeting in ten minutes." When his sandwich arrives, he devours it, while concentrating on the presentation, and washes it down with iced tea, followed by more coffee and a cigarette. Then, to freshen his breath, he pops a stick of gum into his mouth.

An hour and a half later, Warren returns from the meeting to his office. There are telephone messages to be answered and more paperwork to take care of as a result of the meeting. He has indigestion, feels bloated, and has abdominal pain. And no wonder!

It is important to understand that although some foods may be bothersome, it is often the way they are eaten, rather than the specific food, that aggravates symptoms.

Rules to Eat By

Attempt to set aside enough time to eat so that you have the opportunity to dine in an unhurried, relaxed atmosphere. Take time to properly chew your food. Chewing makes the whole remainder of the digestive process easier, allowing your digestive tract to function as it was designed to function. As you may recall, chewing is the only aspect of the digestive process over which you routinely exercise conscious control. (Digestion is unconsciously controlled by the automatic nervous system, which responds to deep-breathing techniques and autohypnosis. See Chapter 9, "Stress and the Intestinal Tract.")

Chances are you would not attempt to place a raw carrot in your stomach without chewing. But even if you are eating well-cooked, puréed carrots, you should still take the time to eat slowly. This allows the digestive enzymes from the salivary glands to mix with the food. Those eating too quickly also often swallow an excessive amount of air (aerophagia), ending up with a bloated feeling. So the first advice to Warren would be to take advantage of this conscious aspect of digestion: eat slowly and chew your food well.

Another word of advice to Warren would be to limit liquid intake with meals—particularly very hot or very cold liquids. Hot liquids may act as a stimulant to the colon, leading to increased cramps. Excessive liquids with a meal may contribute to bloating after a meal, which is often experienced with IBS. Furthermore, some researchers believe that excessive liquid may dilute the digestive enzymes, making them less effective. Other pertinent advice is to avoid carbonated liquids—which contribute to bloating—and to avoid gum or mints after meals. Gum and mints frequently lead to swallowing air, which in turn leads to an uncomfortable distension of the intestine—much like blowing up a balloon. Carbonated beverages, gum, and mints may all contribute to increased intestinal gas. Incidentally, excessive gas and bloating are the most common gastrointestinal complaints.

Research has shown that frequent small meals throughout the day may lead to less discomfort than one or two large ones. Eating frequent small meals means that your system is not overburdened at any one time. Just as an automobile performs more efficiently at a constant speed, your personal "food processor" works more smoothly when you avoid sudden starts and stops.

Eating too quickly often leads to overeating, for several reasons. For one, your food will expand in your stomach as digestive juices are secreted, a process that takes time. Haven't we all eaten too quickly, only to experience that uncomfortable, bloated feeling some 30 minutes or so later? In addition, the hormone cholecystokinin, which is released from the duodenum into the bloodstream in response to a meal, goes to the satiety center in the brain, telling when you've had enough. If you eat too quickly, your body does not have time for this process to occur. As one dietician proclaimed, "I tell my clients to make love to their food…savor each bite."

Caffeine, Alcohol, and Nicotine

In addition to the act of eating, there are three other common triggers of symptoms. Caffeine, alcohol, and nicotine are often referred to as "social drugs." They are, in fact, drugs in every sense of the word, and yet they are socially accepted—although tobacco use is becoming less socially acceptable as users find themselves increasingly ostracized when they indulge in public. As for alcohol and caffeine use, I believe the best

TIPS FOR MEALTIMES

- Whenever possible, make mealtimes a chance to relax.
- Concentrate on chewing thoroughly, and swallowing without haste or gulping air.
- Do not conduct intense business or carry on emotionally charged discussions.
- Arguing or watching disturbing stories on the news while eating may prompt your "food processor" to reject lunch or dinner, leading to acid indigestion.
- Remember, it is often the circumstances surrounding the meal, rather than a specific food, that worsens digestive symptoms.

course—whether or not you have a digestive problem—is using only moderate amounts of these substances, if you do not eliminate them altogether.

Many of my patients find it very difficult to give up coffee when I suggest it. "It gets me going," they say. True. For many, caffeine serves to "jump-start" their engines to overcome the inertia of arising. In this regard, caffeine, which stimulates the central nervous system, acts much like an amphetamine, with its energy-boosting characteristics. Unfortunately, over a period of time, humans can develop a tolerance for caffeine, just as they do with other drugs. What this means is that it may later take two or even three cups of coffee or tea in the morning to "get the engine revving." In addition, as the effects from the initial cups of coffee wear off, a withdrawal period ensues—fatigue sets in, and it takes more coffee or tea periodically throughout the day, to boost the engine level.

Now I am not trying to spoil any pleasure you may derive from caffeinated beverages. I am simply explaining why it may be most difficult for you to give up caffeine, even though you may conclude that it aggravates your digestive problems.

These inherent difficulties stem from the simple fact that caffeine—like other drugs—is addicting, and you may well experience an unpleasant period of withdrawal as you reduce or eliminate your consumption. Symptoms of caffeine withdrawal include decreased energy, irritability, and so-called caffeine-withdrawal headaches.

Many cola drinks also contain caffeine. In addition, caffeine is often an ingredient in noncola carbonated beverages and is sometimes used in over-the-counter pain relief medications. Always check the labels for ingredients or contents. Recent evidence also suggests that many over-the-counter analgesics or pain medications taken on a daily basis may produce "withdrawal headaches." Like caffeine, they may also have an adverse effect on the digestive tract during this withdrawal phase.

At this point, you may be asking yourself, "Why, pray tell, should I give up coffee if giving it up will make me feel this bad?" The fact is that your use of caffeine may be making you feel even worse now and you simply don't realize it. Furthermore, after experiencing a brief period of withdrawal symptoms, you will probably find that you feel better and actually have more energy than you did while you were a caffeine "addict."

Many people depend on caffeine to stimulate a bowel movement in the morning, and it may, in fact, help some people who are prone to constipation "keep regular." However, since caffeine is somewhat of a colonic stimulant, it may well exacerbate the cramp-like abdominal pains and diarrhea experienced by many IBS sufferers. If you rely on caffeine each morning to stimulate a bowel movement, you may find a warm cup of decaffeinated herbal tea works equally well in helping you keep your schedule.

If you are prone to constipation, keep in mind that bowel function is considered to be subject to habit. Therefore, you should allow a period of time at about the same time each day for a bowel movement. I refer to this process as "adult toilet training." Once established, this daily ritual may be more helpful as a colonic stimulant than the morning cup of coffee. Current medical opinion is that many of those who are very constipated are actually blocking out, or unconsciously ignoring, the urge to have a bowel movement. A popular health adage puts it this way:

When Nature calls, don't try to bluff her,
But haste away without delay, or you will surely suffer.

In addition to intensifying the cramps and diarrhea associated with a spastic colon, caffeine has other adverse effects on the digestive system. It may produce inflammation and even cause ulcers to form in the stomach by stimulating increased secretion of stomach acid. Even decaffeinated coffee, like caffeinated coffee, contains tannic acid, which may aggravate ulcer symptoms. In addition, caffeine relaxes the lower esophageal sphincter (LES), the valve between the esophagus and the stomach. This relaxation sometimes allows acid in the stomach to back up into and burn the esophagus, leading to heartburn or acid indigestion.

As a stimulant, caffeine may also worsen anxiety-related symptoms associated with IBS, such as nervousness and palpitations. Incidentally, if you are a female suffering from painful fibrocystic breasts or premenstrual syndrome (PMS), you should avoid all caffeine. See Chapter 16, "Facts About Coexisting Conditions," for a further discussion of PMS. I hope all this evidence will give you reason to eliminate or at least reduce your ingestion of this "social drug."

Another "social drug" is considered to have "medicinal properties" in small amounts. After all, alcohol helps you unwind after a stressful day, and is often found in many cough preparations. However, anyone who has ever experienced a hangover is well acquainted with the consequences of overindulgence. Even drinking what may be considered moderate amounts of alcohol can trigger unpleasant symptoms by impairing the digestion of food present in the intestines, thereby causing gas. Alcohol, like caffeine, may also promote inflammation and ulcers in the stomach. IBS sufferers may find beer particularly bothersome, as this carbonated beverage often contributes to belching, bloating, and excessive gas. If you now use alcohol to help you relax, perhaps it will become less necessary as you learn more about stress and relaxation techniques in Chapter 9. But if you do use alcohol, remember that moderation is the key.

Most people are aware of the deleterious effects that nicotine, particularly cigarette smoking, has on the body. They know that it causes cancer, emphysema, and heart disease. But did you know that it also causes increased secretion of stomach acid and decreased LES pressure, predisposing smokers to heartburn and peptic ulcer disease? Smokers have increased salivation and swallowing as a result of smoke irritation, and they also experience drying of the mucosa lining of the mouth and throat. The phenomenon of air swallowing (aerophagia) mentioned earlier increases air in the stomach and the associated bloated feeling often experienced with IBS. If you are prone to the diarrhea symptoms of IBS, reduction of smoking can help to reduce it. If your spouse smokes, encourage him or her to stop for your benefit as well as his or her own, since the hazardous effects of secondhand smoke are now well known. If you sincerely want to stop smoking, seek the advice of your physician. Also refer to Appendix 4, "How to Stop Smoking," for recommendations on how to reach your goal.

Changing Your Eating Habits

You have learned how to eat and what common IBS triggers to avoid. The next logical question is, what can I eat? Assuming—for the time being—that you have no food sensitivities, or that you are unaware of having any, I recommend the same basic diet for everyone. Food sensitivities are discussed in Chapter 5, "Tracking Down Problem Diet Factors." This "ideal diet" will not only make you less susceptible to IBS but should also help control your weight and give you abundant energy.

You are probably thinking: "This sounds too good to be true. Does this guy believe in the good fairy too?" If you happen to be overweight, you have probably experimented with lots of other diets. An obese patient once told me, "I have lost a thousand pounds over the past fifteen years." Sadly, with dieting, this often happens. Weight is lost only to be regained, then lost again. Personally, I do not like the word "diet," because it conjures up thoughts of deprivation in the minds of those who have been placed—or have placed themselves—on a diet. Deprivation diets invariably lead to feelings of depression, and depression, in turn, leads to failure. The key, then, is to change your eating habits rather than "going on a diet."

There are only two basic requirements to remember if you want to change your eating habits (or make any lifestyle changes, for that matter). These two basic requirements are motivation and knowledge. Pain is a very strong motivational force for many—as an IBS sufferer, this discomfort has obviously motivated you to seek help. You may be further motivated by a desire to lose weight or increase your energy level.

The second requirement—knowledge—provides you with the necessary information to achieve your goal. How much calcium do I need? What vitamins should I take? How can I get more fiber in my diet? These are all questions that my patients frequently ask. Unfortunately, in the area of nutrition, there is an abundance of misinformation. Many patients have told me that the more books they read by so-called nutritional experts, the more confused they become. In addition, whereas current nutritional wisdom places a greater emphasis on increased intake of complex carbohydrates (such as breads, rice, pasta, and beans),

TREATMENT OF IBS: MILD SYMPTOMS

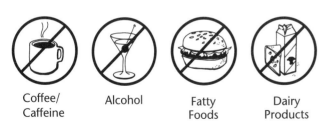

| Coffee/ | Alcohol | Fatty | Dairy |
| Caffeine | | Foods | Products |

Eliminate food and drink that make symptoms worse.

these food were not necessarily emphasized in the past. The reality is that recommendations may change as new facts surface.

The Ideal Diet

Now, having said all that, just what is this "ideal diet" that I recommend? Most people are aware that the average North American diet is much too high in sugar, fats, salt, and protein. As discussed in Chapter 5, a meal with a high fat content may exacerbate IBS symptoms. Excessive sweets and too much protein also seem to worsen symptoms in many people, at least to the extent that these foods take the place of needed complex carbohydrates in the diet. In addition, excessive salt leads to fluid retention, which may contribute to that "bloated" feeling.

So the "ideal diet" should be high in complex carbohydrates (whole grains, fruits, and vegetables), low in fats (particularly saturated fats and cholesterol), with moderate amounts of protein. Limit your intake of sweets and salt. Sounds simple, doesn't it? Actually, proper nutrition is rather simple, but if you are now on the average North American diet, plan to change your eating habits gradually and permanently. You can reduce your intake of sugar, fat, salt, and protein, and learn to relish more healthful alternatives. Dan Reeves, former Denver Broncos football coach, responded, "If it tastes good spit it out," when asked what diet he'd been placed on after a heart attack.

This brings up the next natural question. Is it possible to have palatable, appetizing dishes without salt, rich, creamy sauces, and sugar? I say, unequivocally, YES! Realize that butter, salt, and sugar are actually only flavor enhancers. We just got carried away with their use at some point, as in the cliché "If a little is good, more will be even better." The solution is to try to use the smallest amount possible of these substances to complement any dish you are preparing. Instead, experiment with fresh herbs and spices to enhance flavor.

As a native of Louisiana, I grew up with a passion for good food. I enjoy cooking as a hobby and come from a family of excellent cooks. Through the years in our household, we have learned, largely through experimentation, to prepare wholesome and delicious meals with very small quantities of the traditional flavor enhancers. Make a point of experimenting with new foods and new recipes. The many vegetarian books available now offer recipes for replacing processed foods, sauces, and spices with natural foods that are low in saturated fats and cholesterol. For two excellent sources of nutritional information, read Jane Brody's *Good Food Book* and *Cooking Light*.

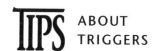

TIPS ABOUT TRIGGERS

Fats and sweets are the most common triggers for IBS symptoms. Decreasing these foods in your diet often leads to significant improvement.

At this point a word about nutritional supplements in general may be appropriate. For years, I felt as many physicians do: that eating a well-balanced diet should provide all the vitamins, minerals, and nutrients the body needs to function at peak performance. However, in recent years I have become convinced from personal experience and reading the literature that this notion may not be correct. Recent studies have demonstrated the beneficial effects of various herbs, vitamins, minerals, and amino acids in disease treatment, prevention and overall well-being. Although not a blanket endorsement, I do feel supplements have their place as part of a total wellness program. (See Chapter 8 for recommendations on nutritional supplements by Dr. Raphael d'Angelo.) However, like medications, use of supplements should be individualized and caution must be exercised as they may occasionally produce their own side effects.

Food Intolerance or Sensitivities

By following the advice in the preceding sections, you may very likely notice a complete or substantial improvement in your symptoms. If not, it may be that a certain food or foods contribute to your continued discomfort. (You may discover these foods by using the elimination diet in Chapter 5.) Or it may be that your continued IBS symptoms result from your gut's response to stress. The concept that certain specific foods may produce IBS symptoms has merit, since, after all, your gut is bombarded with a variety of foods throughout the day. In past years, we did not enjoy the variety of foods that are available today. Many people lived in rural areas and raised or grew most of the foods they consumed. It was much easier to trace problem reactions to foods that were eaten rarely—particularly seasonal foods. Prepackaged foods and food additives were much less prevalent then than now. Today it is difficult to discover if chronic symptoms are occurring in reaction to foods eaten daily—or several times a week—or to ingredients that may be "hidden" within preprocessed preparations. The presence of such hidden foods may help explain the increased prevalence of IBS, or spastic colon, in our affluent society.

The consensus among physicians today is that food indeed plays a part in producing IBS symptoms in a proportion of IBS sufferers. However, opinions differ as to the mechanisms, manifestations, and frequency of food allergies. "Allergy" may not be the most precise term to use when describing the majority of patients whose symptoms worsen when they eat certain foods, since allergy in the true sense of the word usually fails to occur.

With a true allergic reaction, a disruptive interaction occurs between the substance to which you are allergic (the allergen) and your body's preformed antibodies. This process sets into motion a series of events that may cause symptoms, such as wheezing, shortness of breath, hives, flushing, skin rash, and occasionally abdominal cramps and diarrhea. Most people's IBS dietary reactions do not involve the interaction of allergens and antibodies.

That is why we often speak of a "food intolerance," or "food sensitivities." It really is largely a matter of semantics. Call it what you will, certain people experience worsening symptoms with certain foods, and the mechanisms underlying these "reactions" differ. An example of the most common food sensitivity will help explain these concepts.

Juanita was an 18-year-old college freshman I saw some six weeks after her first semester of school. She complained of frequent loose bowel movements, abdominal pains and cramps, and excessive gas. Her bowel movements were more numerous and bothersome just before exams. While obtaining a detailed dietary history, I learned that Juanita had developed a taste for ice cream because the school cafeteria had an ice cream dispenser. I suggested that she eliminate all dairy products for a trial basis of two weeks. During a follow-up visit, she reported an almost complete resolution of her symptoms, except for occasional diarrhea and cramps preceding "big tests." Juanita's major problem, it turns out, was a sensitivity to dairy products, a so-called "lactose intolerance," although she did seem to have a tendency towards the "spastic colon" variety of IBS when she was placed in a stressful situation.

Lactose Intolerance

Dairy products are the foods most likely to produce or exacerbate symptoms. In fact, I have found many patients to have a pure lactose intolerance without the underlying intestinal disorder seen in IBS.

What happens with lactose intolerance? You may recall from the discussion of digestion that your body produces various enzymes that break down large molecules into smaller molecules, which are more easily absorbed by the intestines. Lactose is a complex sugar molecule found in dairy products. Under ordinary circumstances, lactose is broken down into its constituent simple sugars: glucose and galactose. The enzyme responsible for this reaction is found in cells of the small intestine and is called lactase. For reasons that are unclear, as you grow older your body loses the ability to make the lactase enzyme. If your body is unable to digest and absorb lactose, then this complex molecule remains in the intestines, where it is acted upon by normal intestinal bacteria, leading to symptoms of carbohydrate malabsorption—namely, cramps, gas, bloating, and diarrhea.

Does lactose intolerance mean you can never again enjoy dairy products? The answer is no. Fortunately, you may now obtain milk that is treated to be lactose free. You will find that this milk tastes sweeter, since the lactose has already been broken down into its constituent sugars. Alternatively, you can treat milk yourself with over-the-counter lactase enzyme drops to reduce or eliminate its lactase content. Lactase enzyme

TIPS ABOUT LACTOSE INTOLERANCE

- It becomes more common as you grow older.
- It is more common in certain ethnic groups—particularly among people with African or Asian origins.
- Since the lactase enzyme is found in the intestinal cells, an infection of the gastrointestinal tract such as "intestinal flu" may damage these same cells and produce a temporary intolerance of dairy products.
- A hydrogen breath test may be used to determine the presence of lactose intolerance. (See Appendix 2, "Common Questions and Answers About IBS.")

supplements are also available; when taken with dairy products, these aid in digestion and the absorption of lactose. (See Appendix 3 for a lactose-free diet.)

If you elect to avoid all dairy products, I strongly recommend that you consider taking a supplement with calcium and vitamin D to prevent later development of osteoporosis, particularly if you are female. There are multiple calcium supplements on the market. I recommend calcium citrate because studies indicate that it is better absorbed than other calcium supplements. The usual recommended intake of calcium is 1000 to 1500 milligrams per day. In North America, approximately 60 percent of the daily intake of calcium is derived from milk and other dairy products. Other sources of calcium include meats, certain fish, and green, leafy vegetables.

Nowadays lactose intolerance is common and easily recognized by most physicians. However, it was not understood until 1965. Before that time, those with pure lactose intolerance would have been lumped together with others considered to have IBS. It may turn out that as our present understanding of IBS increases, we may discover still other enzyme deficiencies that appear to cause IBS symptoms.

Sugar Reactions

Large amounts of sugar are not digested well by anyone, much less someone with IBS. The naturally occurring sugars, fructose and sorbitol, produce effects similar to those seen with lactose intolerance. Fructose is found in fruits and berries as well as onions, artichokes, pears, and wheat. It is also used as a sweetener in many fruit drinks and soft drinks (for example, "high-fructose corn syrup"). Sorbitol is found in fruits, including apples, pears, peaches, and prunes; it is also used as an artificial sweetener in many "sugar-free" or dietetic products.

I have seen countless IBS patients benefit from the recommendation that they decrease their intake of soft drinks when fructose intolerance was felt to be an underlying factor. One physician has dubbed the term "Halloween diarrhea" to describe children who develop abdominal bloating and diarrhea after consuming large amounts of sorbitol in candy during times of increased ingestion, such as Halloween.

Citrus fruits and juices may also worsen symptoms, presumably by increasing the sugar load and acid load (citric acid) in the intestinal tract. Be wary of the current "juicing" craze as this process serves to concentrate higher amounts of fructose, unmasking a previously unrecognized fructose intolerance. The same phenomenon can occur when juicing with vegetables as well. It takes approximately three oranges to make a small glass of orange juice. You would be much better off eating the orange and drinking a glass of water with it. Most juicers do not retain the beneficial fiber in the final product.

Gas-forming Foods

The production of gas is a normal physiologic function, and probably the most common gastrointestinal complaint. It is caused by several factors, one of which is food. While IBS sufferers do not have more gas than others, they may be more sensitive to it, and would do well to avoid foods that cause them gas.

Gas results when naturally occurring bacteria in the large intestine digest complex carbohydrates—starches, fiber, and sugars. Complex carbohydrates cause the most gas, whereas proteins and fats cause little gas. There are four types of sugars that cause gas—lactose, fructose, sorbitol (discussed earlier), and raffinose, which is found in the cruciferous vegetables, such as broccoli, cabbage, cauliflower, brussels sprouts, and beans. Many of my patients find that cucumbers frequently cause belching and gas. The cruciferous vegetables are often better digested when well cooked or puréed in a soup. You may also consider using BEANO, an oral enzyme supplement that helps to break down the complex carbohydrates in cruciferous vegetables and beans. Many of my patients find it a valuable supplement, allowing them to enjoy healthy foods that may also help reduce the incidence of colon cancer.

The following chapter will help you to identify all the foods that may be problematic to you. In Chapter 15, "Treating Recurring Symptoms," I explain further how gas is caused and can be prevented.

Food Additives

The role food additives play in producing IBS symptoms is just beginning to be explored. However, the relationship of food additives to other disorders is already clear: sulfites have a negative effect on asthma, and monosodium glutamate (MSG) may precipitate migraine headaches. Sulfites are used as a preservative in the processing of wine and beer and in restaurants to maintain the crispness of fruits and vegetables (commonly where salad bars exist). MSG is used as a flavor enhancer in many packaged, processed, and frozen foods.

To determine if MSG is a trigger for IBS symptoms, I conducted a study from 1994 to 1996, with a grant from the Presbyterian/St. Luke's Foundation. We studied diarrhea-predominant IBS patients, excluding those whose IBS symptoms were solely aggravated by stress. In this "double-blind cross-over trial," patients were given a meal with MSG, and at a different time, a similar meal without MSG; neither they nor the investigators knew which meal contained the MSG. The results of this study indicated that there was an association between MSG ingestion and abdominal pain in a group of IBS sufferers we studied. Symptoms not related to IBS but known to be associated with MSG sensitivity—headache, muscle tightness, flushing, and dizziness—were also experienced to a significant degree by those who ate the meal with the additive.

Controversy has surrounded the use of MSG over the past 30 years due to reports of adverse reactions to the additive. The FDA believes that MSG and related substances are safe for most people when eaten at customary levels. However, it recognizes that some people may have MSG sensitivity. The grassroots movement Truth in Labeling says that in MSG-sensitive people, the additive causes a wide range of adverse reactions affecting not only the gastrointestinal tract, but also the heart and circulatory system, muscles, skin, vision, and neurological and urological systems.

Technically speaking, MSG is a sodium salt of glutamic acid that has been freed from the protein during the manufacturing process. (It appears that it is the "free" glutamic acid produced, and not the protein—glutamic acid—that causes adverse reactions.) Another way of describing this manufacturing process is "hydrolyzing." Hydrolyzed proteins or protein hydrolysates are used in the same manner as MSG in many foods, such as canned vegetables, soups, and processed meats. The FDA says that foods containing hydrolyzed proteins have relatively high levels of free glutamate, ranging from 5 to 20 percent.

Currently, common food ingredients such as tomatoes used for tomato paste and hydrolyzed soy protein used for soy sauce contain free glutamates as natural constituents, and as such, are not listed on labels. (Also, incidental additives used in processing that are considered insignificant amounts and without a technical or functional effect in the finished food are not listed in labels.) But the FDA does recognize that some people are sensitive to free glutamates, and is considering a labeling policy respecting glutamate-intolerance. For a list of foods containing MSG and free glutamic acid, see Chapter 5.

Individuals with a known glutamate sensitivity are also usually sensitive to aspartic acid, which is the main constituent of aspartame (the artificial sweetener in Nutrasweet). Glutamic acid and aspartic acid share common receptors and are so-called neuroexcitatory amino acids. Neuroexcitatory amino acids "excite" the taste buds by stimulating nerves which mediate the sensation of taste. In susceptible individuals they may stimulate nerves in the brain and elsewhere, resulting in undesirable side effects.

Olestra (or its brand name Olean) is another food additive that may also cause IBS symptoms. It is a fat substitute made from vegetable oils and sugar but is not digested and therefore not consumed as calories. However, because it is not digested, it may irritate the bowels and cause IBS symptoms.

Until we understand more about the role of food additives and IBS, you would do well to remember the motto of Boston's Bread & Circus Whole Food Supermarkets and try to eat only "the food, the whole food, and nothing but the food."

CHAPTER 5

Tracking Down
Problem Diet Factors

B Y NOW, you will have begun to see the picture: your diet may affect the way you feel, and everyone's digestive system is unique. The diet that is trouble- free for you may not be so for someone else.

We all have subtle dietary nuances that make us individuals. How we eat, what we eat, and when we eat may all play a part in intensifying IBS symptoms in susceptible persons. The most common foods thought to induce sensitivities include fats and sweets, dairy products, wheat, cruciferous vegetables, citrus fruits and fruit juices, chocolate, and eggs. Sweets and meals with a high fat content are troublesome for many people. Suffering from IBS does not necessarily mean you will react negatively to any or all of the above; nor does this list include all foods that have been linked with sensitivities. So how do you track down any special food sensitivities you may have?

The Importance of Using a Diet Diary

You must assume an active role if you wish to track down any complicating factors that may contribute to your IBS symptoms, and you must be introspective. A diet diary is the chief tool to help you achieve this goal. All you need is commitment, a pen or pencil, and a notebook.

First, record what you ate and when. You may want to record your diet diary in a notebook and base it on the example below, or you may want to copy and use the sample diet diary. Either way, you may follow the instructions for keeping a diet diary in this chapter. When keeping your diary, be as specific as you can regarding quantities and types of food (including brand names)—remember the hidden ingredients in many preprocessed foods. For example, an entry might read:

11:30 a.m.—1 tablespoon of Brand X Chunky Peanut Butter, with two tablespoons of Brand X Strawberry Preserves, and two slices of Brand X Bread (white).

Such an entry will give you much more valuable information for later analysis than simply writing down:

Lunch—peanut butter and jelly sandwich.

It is also important to record foods in the order you ate them, since you may find you cannot tolerate some foods on an empty stomach, whereas the same foods may be safely eaten with other foods.

Don't forget to list all condiments and liquids, including types of water, you consume. For example:

1 tablespoon of butter, 2 tablespoons of Brand X Italian dressing, 12 oz. Brand X diet cola.

In addition include the type of day you are having:

Rushing, late for work, relaxing day at the beach, etc. Note the stress level ratings on the sample diet diary and circle the appropriate number corresponding to your range of stress levels on that day. List any exercise or physical activity that exceeds your usual activities of daily living.

Finally, record the type and timing of any symptoms you experience:

8:00 a.m.—Feeling nauseous.

2:30 p.m.—Bloated, excessive gas.

The diet diary is a tool to help you and your doctor analyze and become aware of your daily food habits and choices. It works best if you fill it out immediately after eating or drinking. The diet diary is most helpful when kept daily. If you tend to eat more on weekends or social occasions, make sure to note those days and occasions in the diary.

I suggest keeping your diary at least two weeks before attempting to determine if there are any patterns. Obviously, the longer you keep your diet diary, the more helpful it will be, particularly if you go out for, say, Chinese food only once a month. When eating out, make a note of the restaurant you dined in, and inquire about the contents of any sauces, stuffing, or casseroles. I have two patients who can tolerate all types of seafood with the single exception of scallops. They must be careful when ordering seafood combinations, as scallops may have been used in the recipe.

Your diet diary will help you become a medical detective, so you may be able to later eliminate or reduce the offending agents in your diet. Many of my patients return to me to review their diet diaries, and during this process they are able to determine the specific food groups and circumstances that worsen their symptoms. You may find that pizza and beer during Monday night football is a no-no. You may also find that your symptoms are related more to your stress level on a given day than to any specific foods. Or you may discover that on days you skip breakfast and lunch and have a large dinner late in the evening your symptoms are particularly bad. In addition, many overweight patients who take the time to record food intake are surprised by how much they actually eat, and use their diet diary as an aid to reducing calories.

Periodically, retest your system to refine and amend the list of foods to which you experience an adverse reaction.

DIET DIARY

NAME:_____

DATE:_____

Time	Food	Amount	Symptoms	Stress Level: 1 2 3 4 5 (low—high)	Exercise

TIPS ON DIET TRACKING

As you begin the elimination diet, do not take the negative approach: "I can eat hardly anything." Rather, emphasize the positive—what you can eat! The goal is to determine what foods you can tolerate, and the reward will be the security of knowing there are foods you can enjoy without troublesome symptoms.

The Elimination Diet—A Thorough and Complex Approach

The elimination, or exclusion, diet is an alternative and more precise approach to tracking down your food sensitivities. This procedure, though sometimes necessary, is more involved than keeping a diet diary and looking for patterns. And since it could require a restrictive diet for an extended period, during it your body may not receive all the nutrients it requires. Therefore, I recommend the use of an elimination diet only while under the supervision of a physician or nutritionist. Dr. K. W. Heaton, who presented a paper at the 1995 International Symposium on Functional Gastrointestinal Disorders, states, "Elimination diets should be part of the repertoire of every physician who treats patients with intractable irritable bowel syndrome." Such a diet is not intended to deprive or punish you, but rather to help you gain peace of mind in knowing what foods you can tolerate, and to help you identify those that clearly are problematic.

Basically, the exclusion diet consists of eliminating certain foods from your diet and then gradually reintroducing those food groups and charting your body's reaction. This reintroduction of food groups is called "rechallenging" and is discussed in greater detail later in this chapter.

Fortunately, food intolerance is not very complex in the majority of cases. In isolated instances, however, it may be necessary to sharpen your detective skills if you still suffer symptoms after following the advice so far in this book. For example, suppose you have taken care to eat slowly, chewing food well and in a relaxed atmosphere; you have eliminated caffeine, alcohol, and nicotine; you have modified your present diet to more closely resemble the "ideal diet"; and you have experimented with avoiding such common triggers as dairy products, wheat, fats, and sweets. If you have followed all of these recommendations and are still having problems, then it may become necessary to try an elimination diet. Because diarrhea and gas are more frequently complaints of those with food reactions, if these symptoms persist an exclusion diet is the best tool for determining whether you have a food intolerance or sensitivity.

Stress as another factor in the development of IBS symptoms is discussed in detail later. You need to be ever aware of both emotional and physiological stress as a trigger of symptoms so as not to wrongly implicate a particular food. With this idea in mind, you will also realize the importance of periodically retesting certain foods, to see if they must remain on your restricted list. Stress may be one of several factors that make food intolerance seem to be intermittent. Some food intolerances develop over time. For example, lactose intolerance becomes more common with advancing age; others may occur temporarily, such as after a bout of gastroenteritis or a course of antibiotics.

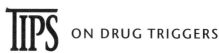

TIPS ON DRUG TRIGGERS

Pay attention to the effects of medications when tracking down problem factors. Use the diet diary and note any IBS symptoms when you are taking antibiotics, high blood pressure medications, diuretics, or narcotics—all may cause or worsen the symptoms of IBS. For example, prescription cough preparations and pain medications can cause constipation.

If you suspect that just a few foods are causing a reaction, you need eliminate only those foods. For example, lactose intolerance is diagnosed by eliminating dairy products from your diet for a specified time. If your symptoms disappear during testing, rechallenge your digestive system at a later date to see if symptoms reappear.

It is best to use the simplest form of the substance when retesting your system. For example, when retesting for dairy product intolerance, drink a glass of milk rather than eating a bowl of ice cream. Ice cream also contains sugar, heavy cream, eggs, and flavorings and additives, all of which may confuse your diagnosis. Milk consists of three main ingredients: sugar (lactose), protein (casein), and fat. Lactose is the most likely culprit when individuals react negatively to milk. Rarely, we see a true protein "allergy" to casein, and the fat content of milk will bother some, but they can drink skim milk without difficulty.

One of my more mature IBS patients had given up milk with his morning cereal feeling he was lactose intolerant. Further detective work and a switch from whole milk to skim milk proved it was really the fat content of the whole milk causing his symptoms. "I never thought I could develop a taste for skim milk," he proudly exclaimed on a follow-up visit.

As a further example, when retesting for wheat sensitivity, obtain a whole wheat cereal without sugar or additives, rather than whole wheat bread, which may contain other ingredients, such as sugar and yeast. Gluten is a wheat protein found within the wheat kernel. Wheat bran is the outer coating of the wheat kernel. Many people who are intolerant of whole wheat products are reacting to the gluten but may tolerate the wheat bran. Conversely, some people can tolerate refined white flour and react to whole wheat products, suggesting a sensitivity to the outer bran coat of the wheat kernel. I am really not trying to confuse you; I am simply using these examples to point out some of the complexities of food intolerance.

"Aren't there any tests you can perform to determine which foods I am allergic to?" is a question I am frequently asked. Unfortunately, the few tests available are of limited use. Skin tests and the RAST (radioallergosorbent test) will identify those rare individuals with true allergies to certain foods, in which the body has preformed antibodies to a particular food—milk protein or casein, for example. It will not detect the more common food intolerances, such as lactose intolerance, which is the result of enzyme deficiency. From a practical point of view, using an elimination diet remains the most effective way to discover your food intolerances.

To my knowledge, there is no single exclusion diet that is generally accepted and that can be used by everyone following a course for dietary manipulation. In fact, many physicians who treat IBS downplay the contribution of food intolerance. This position is defensible, because making common-sense dietary changes and avoiding common, well-established IBS triggers will usually be enough.

Specialists in gastroenterology and those physicians with a special interest in treating IBS generally see the tougher cases, referred to them after the usual therapeutic approaches have failed. For them an exclusion diet may be very useful, unless, of course, the physician suspects emotional or other factors such as adverse reactions to medications, or even a different diagnosis. One study reported that symptoms improved in 48 percent of patients placed on an exclusion diet for three weeks. The patients were chosen for the study because they had not improved with "conventional therapy." However, this study did not address the multiplicity of mechanisms underlying food intolerances.

Food additives, for example, are not commonly considered for exclusion diets. Ralph, a 40-year-old businessman, came to see me complaining of intermittent cramps and abdominal pain. He traveled frequently, but kept a regular schedule for rest and meals at restaurants, and appeared to have a healthy diet. We decided a diet diary would help to track down a possible food intolerance or trigger. After two weeks his diary showed that Ralph's IBS symptoms improved, but then returned when we challenged his system by adding MSG to his diet. Many patients I see with MSG sensitivity also experience a myriad of other symptoms, including common complaints such as headache, inability to concentrate, and muscular aching similar to fibromyalgia syndrome (see Chapter 16, "Facts About Coexisting Conditions").

 ON MSG TRIGGERS

If you suspect a MSG or glutamate sensitivity:
- Avoid prepackaged or processed foods—chicken bouillon and low-fat salad dressings are particularly problematic.
- Learn the names of other food additives that contain MSG.
- Read labels!
- Eat fresh fruits, fresh vegetables, and fresh meats.

Foods to avoid when following an elimination diet, together with those foods generally allowed, are listed below. I have compiled this information based on a review of the literature on food intolerance and IBS, as well as my own experience in treating this disorder. Some physicians may think that this list is too restrictive, whereas others may find it not restrictive enough, and I again caution you to use the exclusion diet only under the supervision of a physician or registered dietitian. I also advise you to closely adhere to the following points while on the exclusion diet:

- Never eat a food that may have caused a life-threatening reaction in the past, even if that food is on the list of allowed foods.

- Exclude any foods from the following "Foods Allowed" list that you have previously identified or suspected as a cause of symptoms.
- When possible, and under the direction of your physician, avoid all nonessential medications, whether prescription or over-the-counter. Otherwise, what you suspect to be a reaction may actually be a side effect caused by the medication.
- Stay on the exclusion diet for a period of two weeks. During this time, eat only the foods allowed. If you are not prepared to strictly adhere to the diet, do not waste your time. Any variation will invalidate the results, requiring you to start all over again.
- Read all labels carefully! Many foods or substances on the list to avoid may be hidden in prepackaged or processed food products. Whenever possible, eat fresh, "whole foods" in an unadulterated state. By avoiding prepackaged and processed foods, you may discover if you have any sensitivity to food additives. (See Chapter 7, "Nutrition and Meal Planning," for more information about food labels.)
- Remember that food intolerance or sensitivity is often quantitative as well as qualitative. In other words, small amounts of a certain food "trigger" may not produce negative symptoms, but once the amount exceeds a certain threshold, symptoms will occur. Furthermore, some troublesome foods may only produce negative symptoms when eaten alone and yet are tolerated as part of a meal.
- As you begin, keep a diet diary, as discussed earlier in this chapter. If your symptoms have not improved at all within two weeks, then it is unlikely that food intolerance is a factor, and you should consult your physician regarding other approaches to your treatment. If symptoms improve, you may begin the reintroduction phase of the diet.
- Begin your exclusion diet when your life is stable and free of new activities or special stresses. However, be careful not to procrastinate by waiting too long for a stress-free starting date.

Retesting Your System

Assuming that your symptoms have improved on the elimination diet, it is now time to determine which of the eliminated foods or food groups may have been causing a problem. It is hoped that there will be enough foods you enjoy on the "Foods Allowed" list to give you a nutritious "emergency diet" to fall back on when symptoms flare. You should always have enough "safe foods" on hand, whether at home or while traveling, to help you through a rough time. Your personal list of foods allowed should grow as you reintroduce and discover the foods you can tolerate from the "Foods to Avoid" list.

There are several important points to bear in mind when retesting food groups:

- The reaction to a particular food may be considerably delayed. Therefore, wait to reintroduce new foods every three days.
- Keep track of what you ate, when you ate it, and your symptoms, if any, in your diet diary.
- Keep your meal patterns consistent, preferably eating several small meals during the day, such as three meals with healthful snacks in between meals.
- Eat adequate amounts, at least two or three servings a day, of the foods to be tested, in their most basic forms. For example, drink lots of milk when testing dairy products, rather than eating ice cream or cheese. If no symptoms occur after three days, add this food to your "Foods Allowed" list.
- If you have a negative reaction with reintroduction of a food, put it on the "Foods to Avoid" list. Then wait until you are completely symptom free before resuming testing with another food group.
- Plan to retest, at a later date, those foods that seem to initially cause a problem. If, after several such trials, you find a food consistently causes problems, add that food to your "Foods to Avoid" list.
- Review your findings with your doctor or dietitian to ensure that your list of allowed foods is nutritionally adequate.

I usually recommend initial retesting with dairy products, although the order in which you reintroduce foods from the "Foods to Avoid" list is not important. Many patients have a good idea of whether or not they tolerate dairy products before they even begin the elimination diet. I suggest first trying skim, rather than whole, milk. This will prevent confusing a negative reaction to milk fat (found in whole milk) with symptoms due to lactose intolerance. If you have no reaction to skim milk, you may assume that you do not have lactose intolerance. If the issue still remains unclear, you may wish to try the hydrogen breath test (see Appendix 2, "Common Questions and Answers About IBS") to accurately assess whether you have lactose intolerance. Over the next few days, reintroduce two percent milk, whole milk, low-fat cheese, and other dairy products.

Next, experiment with the various grains, beginning with wheat. Try a whole wheat cereal, which you may eat with milk, if milk is now on the "Foods Allowed" list. Eat wheat bread if you find that yeast is not a problem. Wheat may take longer to produce adverse effects, so test wheat products for at least four days. Gradually reintroduce other grains, such as corn, oats, and barley.

Then begin testing with cooked whole eggs, citrus foods, and various vegetables. Remember, cooked vegetables may be better tolerated. If a particular vegetable (say, broccoli) causes no problems when cooked, you may try it raw later.

It is prudent to minimize your intake of alcohol, caffeine, sweets, and fats, even though they may not cause a specific problem related to IBS. As I am sure you are aware, these substances should be used in moderation for various other health reasons.

Hopefully, the list of problem foods that you identify will be short. Keep an open mind and a positive outlook, and experiment with new foods that you might add to your list of allowed foods.

FOODS TO AVOID AND FOODS ALLOWED
IN AN ELIMINATION DIET

Remember that for most people with IBS, eliminating fats and sweets, gas-forming foods, and caffeine will be adequate. Those with severe symptoms need to pay attention to the following in tracking down problem foods.

Foods to Avoid

Milk and dairy products
This includes cheese, margarine, butter, yogurt, ice cream, many pastries, many candies, and any food containing milk or milk products.

Grains
Wheat, corn, oats, barley, and rye. This includes any product made from or containing wheat flour. This also includes any product that contains corn, cornmeal, or corn oil, and products made from oat or rye flour.

Eggs
This includes any of the countless processed foods that contain eggs, such as ice cream, pastries, salad dressings, and pasta.

Citrus fruits
Oranges, lemons, limes, grapefruits, and beverages containing citrus juice. Most common reactions to other types of fruit are rare.

Vegetables
The cruciferous vegetables broccoli, cabbage, brussels sprouts, and onions cause gas. Turnips, potatoes, asparagus, artichokes, cucumbers, green peppers, and radishes may also cause gas.

Legumes
All beans and peas can cause gas.

Sweets
All foods with a high content of various sugars (the names of these sugars usually end in "ose"), such as sucrose, glucose, fructose, galactose, lactose, and the dietetic sweetener sorbitol, corn syrup, honey, and molasses.

Meats and fish
Cured meats with MSG, bacon, sausage and luncheon meats, smoked fish and shellfish.

Caffeine
All coffee (even decaffeinated, since the acid content of coffee is high enough to cause problems). Avoid all caffeine-containing teas, sodas, and chocolate.

Alcohol
All alcoholic beverages. Beer and wine may be especially problematic. Initially, nonalcoholic malt beverages should also be avoided.

Food Additives
Prepackaged or processed foods often contain food additives, which are not always identified on the labels. Avoid aspartame, olestra, and MSG (monosodium glutamate). Also avoid free

glutamates in the form of hydrolyzed protein, hydrolyzed oat flour, sodium casseinate, yeast extract, yeast nutrient, autolyzed yeast, yeast food, maltodextrin, textured protein, calcium casseinate, malt extract, malt flavoring, bouillon, barley malt, broth, stock, various poultry flavorings and seasonings.

Miscellaneous
Spicy foods, fatty foods, fried foods, salty foods, creamy sauces, yeast-containing foods, and carbonated beverages.

Foods Allowed
Beverages
Tap water, bottled and filtered water (without carbonation), caffeine-free herbal teas, apple juice diluted with water.

Bread and crackers
Only wheat-free and gluten-free bread and crackers, made without yeast or milk products. Try products made with rice flour (rice cakes or rice crackers). Consider baking your own bread using rice flour or flours marked "gluten free," such as arrowroot and tapioca. You may need to visit a health food store to find suitable wheat-free alternatives.

Grains
Rice (preferably brown), puffed-rice cereals, without sugar or additives.

Grains such as millet, amaranth, and quinoa may be well tolerated by gluten-sensitive individuals.

Vegetables
All vegetables not included on the "Foods to Avoid" list. Cooked vegetables may be better tolerated (organic produce is preferable where available).

Legumes
Peas and beans are better tolerated if cooked to a purée and eaten with a digestive enzyme such as BEANO.

Fruits
All other fruits not included on the "Foods to Avoid" list. Cooked, peeled, or unsprayed fruits may be better tolerated. Apples, peaches, and pears may cause gas, and excessive amounts of fruits and vegetables may cause gas and/or diarrhea.

Meats and fish
Of all the meats, fresh chicken and lamb are least likely to cause a problem. Turkey, beef, and pork are allowed. Choose a small portion and a lean cut of meat. Stick with the lighter, less fatty fish with white meat such as halibut, flounder, and sole.

Miscellaneous
Homemade soups and stews made from allowed ingredients are very nutritious.

CHAPTER 6

Discovering the Value of High Fiber

For DECADES, many professionals have advocated an increase in dietary fiber as the cornerstone of IBS treatment. Fiber is the undigested portion of fruits, vegetables, and grains. However, conflicting reports have emerged from time to time regarding the efficacy of fiber in treating IBS. The addition of fiber seems most useful with those IBS sufferers who have a low dietary intake of fiber and a tendency towards constipation (defined by small hard stools that are difficult to pass). There has been a resurgence of interest in using dietary fiber for the prevention and treatment of a wide variety of diseases, including diverticulitis, colorectal cancer, chronic constipation, diabetes, and elevated cholesterol.

Is this simply another food fad? Absolutely not! It is easy to understand the resurgence of interest in increased dietary fiber when we realize that in countries where the intake is high, the incidence of all the disorders mentioned above is correspondingly low, suggesting a possible link. In addition, before the 1900s—when people ate whole foods rather than the refined foods of today—these same diseases were much less prevalent.

Chapter 4, "What You Should Know About Diet," pointed out the importance of increasing your intake of complex carbohydrates (fruits, vegetables, grains). Such a diet, which is high in complex carbohydrates, is also an excellent source of natural dietary fiber.

What Dietary Fiber Does

Dietary fiber is not a single food substance. Fiber is a collective term describing a variety of plant substances that are resistant to digestion by gastrointestinal enzymes. During the time fiber-rich substances remain in the intestinal tract, they produce a number of beneficial effects.

From a mechanical standpoint, fiber adds bulk to the stools, thereby actually helping to reduce the intestinal pressure needed to move intestinal contents along. Fiber also retains water in the stool and increases the propulsive activity of the intestines, which promotes elimination.

In contrast, a diet high in refined carbohydrates has been stripped of most or all of the naturally occurring fiber. These refined carbohydrates—or so-called simple sugars—are almost completely digested and absorbed. What remains in the intestines is only a small amount of residue, creating small, hard stools, which require an increase in intestinal pressure at each bowel movement. The net result may well be constipation and cramps.

From a metabolic standpoint, complex carbohydrates increase energy level, help stabilize blood glucose, and help reduce blood cholesterol. These beneficial metabolic effects explain how high-fiber complex carbohydrates work to prevent diabetes (excess sugar in the blood) and arteriosclerosis (hardening of the arteries). The following examples show how these beneficial effects occur.

The complex carbohydrates found in high-fiber foods must be chemically broken down into smaller molecules before they can be absorbed as simple carbohydrates. This procedure takes time, and calories are actually burned up in the process. This helps to explain complaints of "I am cold all of the time" in those who generally skip breakfast and whose intake of complex carbohydrates is correspondingly low. Eating a breakfast rich in complex carbohydrates is like adding extra wood to the glowing embers of a fire that has been allowed to die down overnight.

The simple carbohydrate glucose is a small molecule and is the major source of the body's energy. When complex carbohydrates are eaten, they slowly break down and are transformed into glucose through a series of metabolic reactions. At the same time, blood glucose gradually

68

rises and falls again. But when you eat something consisting mainly of refined carbohydrates—such as a doughnut made of bleached flour and topped with a sugar glaze—your blood glucose will rise rapidly, and your body will bypass the usual metabolic reactions. This may give you a sudden boost of "quick energy." However, as with many other things in life, you pay a price for this "quick energy," as the body overreacts to this higher-than-normal blood sugar by pouring out insulin from the pancreas in an attempt to decrease the blood glucose. Often the body overshoots, and the extra insulin secreted eventually leads to the symptoms of hypoglycemia or low blood sugar—mainly headache, fatigue, nausea, and nervousness. If you are wondering why the body does not do a better job of regulating such things as blood sugar, it is because your body will work more efficiently if you consume the fuels provided by nature in their original state. After all, have you ever seen a candy bar growing on a tree?

The Different Types of Fiber

Fiber consists of six subtly different substances. Basically, the components of fiber are divided into two groups: those that are soluble in water (pectins, gums and mucilages, and some hemicelluloses), and those that are insoluble in water (lignins, cellulose, and the remainder of the hemicelluloses).

Fruits, vegetables, and grains are not composed exclusively of either soluble or insoluble fibers but contain various amounts of these different compounds. One example of a largely water-insoluble source of fiber is wheat bran, which consists mainly of cellulose and hemicellulose. In contrast, water-soluble fibers have a tendency to retain more water. Some examples of these are bananas and apples, with their high content of pectins. Oat bran, which has received considerable attention recently, is another source of water-soluble fiber.

Water-soluble fibers are also acted upon more than insoluble fibers by bacteria in the colon, through a process known as fermentation. The fermentation process is thought to be important to the formation of an easily passed, moist, bulky stool. Beans, which have a high content of

TIPS ABOUT THE DAILY REQUIREMENT OF FIBER

The average North American consumes approximately 15 to 20 grams of fiber daily. Most nutritionists recommend twice this amount—30 to 40 grams—as beneficial in preventing those conditions that may result from too little dietary fiber. Some nutritional experts recommend adjusting total fiber intake according to total amount of calories consumed. For example, it may be difficult to consume 30 to 40 grams of fiber if you are on a 1,500-calorie diet for weight control, or if your caloric requirements are low. In these cases, 12 grams per 1,000 calories may be a more appropriate recommendation.

gums, are an excellent source of water-soluble fibers. Unfortunately, as you are probably well aware, beans often give rise to distention and excessive gas. If this is a problem for you, you might try the dietary supplement BEANO. Bloating and gas, in turn, may worsen existing bowel symptoms. The key to increasing dietary fiber, without negative side effects worsening an irritable bowel, is to increase your intake of high-fiber foods gradually. Remember, start low and go slow! Your system will generally adjust over a period of time. Also recall that everyone's digestive tract is a bit different, so trial and error may become necessary to find and eliminate those foods that are most disruptive to your digestive system. For example, I have one patient who tolerates most fresh fruits. However, she has found that plums tend to worsen her symptoms, possibly due to their high sorbitol content.

The table, "Foods High in Fiber," should give you some sense of the fiber content of various fruits, vegetables, and grains. Try to obtain your daily fiber requirement by including a variety of foods from this list in your diet. If you are unable to achieve this goal, perhaps temporarily, because of travel away from home, or chronically, as the result of negative reactions to high-fiber foods, you may be able to complement your diet with one of the many fiber supplements available at drugstores, health food stores, and supermarkets. Most of these come in powder form, which, when mixed with the appropriate amount of water, are taken around mealtimes. In this way, the supplement is allowed to mix with the food, helping to provide for soft, formed stools. Psyllium, a water-soluble fiber derived by grinding up seeds from the plantago plant, is the most common ingredient in fiber supplements. It may be found, reasonably priced, in food stores using bulk containers.

FOODS HIGH IN FIBER

This list gives the approximate fiber content of some common high-fiber foods. Use it as a guide to familiarize yourself with foods to include in your diet to achieve the desired intake of 30 to 40 grams of dietary fiber. Remember to increase your intake of dietary fiber gradually so that your intestinal tract can adjust, preventing excessive gas and bloating.

FOOD SOURCE	DIETARY FIBER (GRAMS)
Grains and Breakfast Cereals	
Corn Flakes, ¾ cup	2.0
Puffed Wheat, ¾ cup	1.4
Raisin Bran, ¾ cup	1.0
Shredded Wheat, 1 large biscuit	2.7
Rice, ½ cup cooked brown	2.4
Rice, ½ cup cooked white	0.1
Breads and Crackers	
Rye crackers, 6	2.0
Rye bread, 1 slice	1.0
White bread, 1 slice	0.5
Whole wheat bread, 1 slice	1.4
Fruits	
Apple, 1 medium	2.8
Banana, 1 medium	1.8
Berries, ½ cup	2.0
Cherries, 15 large	1.0
Figs, 2 dried, small	6.4
Grapes, 16	2.0
Orange, 1 medium	3.2
Peach, 1 medium	2.2
Pineapple, ¾ cup	0.5
Plums, 2 medium	1.5
Prunes, 8 large	2.0
Strawberries, 10 large	2.0

FOOD SOURCE	DIETARY FIBER (GRAMS)
Nuts	
Brazil nuts, ¼ cup	2.5
Filberts, ¼ cup	5.0
Peanuts, ¼ cup	3.3
Sunflower seeds, ¼ cup	4.0
Vegetables	
Asparagus, ¾ cup	3.1
Baked beans, 1/3 cup	6.0
Beans, ½ cup pinto	5.3
Beans, ½ cup white	5.0
Beans, ½ cup green	2.1
Beans, ½ cup kidney	5.8
Beets, ½ cup	2.5
Broccoli tops, ½ cup	3.0
Brussels sprouts, ½ cup	2.8
Cabbage, ½ cup	2.8
Cauliflower, ½ cup	1.8
Lettuce, ½ cup	0.5
Onion, ½ cup	2.1
Carrots, ½ cup	3.0
Peas, ½ cup	5.0
Popcorn, 1 cup popped	0.5
Potato, 1 med. baked	3.0
Spinach, ½ cup boiled	5.7
Tomatoes, 1 small	1.4
Turnips, 2/3 cup	2.0
Sweet corn, ½ cup	4.7
Zucchini squash, ½ cup	2.7

Fiber supplements are best taken at mealtimes. I recommend that people who are overweight take fiber supplements before mealtimes so that their appetites may be somewhat curbed. Remember that these supplements contain only fiber; they do not contain the variety of minerals and vitamins found in fruits, vegetables, and grains. Therefore, if you use these products in place of fruits, vegetables, and grains to obtain adequate fiber, check with your doctor regarding the possible need for vitamin and mineral supplements. In addition, make sure the fiber supplements do not contain sugar or artificial sweeteners such as aspartame.

Although controversial, some experts believe that fiber supplements can "normalize" the alternating diarrhea and constipation seen with IBS. During the constipated phase, the water-retaining properties of the fiber allow for a softer stool, whereas during the diarrheal phase, the extra water is absorbed, making the stool firmer. There is certainly more consensus regarding the use of dietary fiber in the treatment of constipation-predominant IBS symptoms.

CHAPTER 7

Nutrition and Meal Planning

Good planning is the key to digestive health. Most agree that to gain financial independence, you must develop a sound financial plan. In fact, the number of financial planners has skyrocketed in recent years. This trend is driven, in part, by the fact that financial security is a comforting and much-pursued goal. I have begun many of my talks on health with development of this concept. "But," you may argue, "this is a book on digestion. What does it have to do with financial planning?" Well, I have found this concept useful in illustrating two points:

• First, a sound, well-conceived plan will increase the likelihood of success in any endeavor.

• Second, financial well-being will be of no value if your personal state of health does not allow you to enjoy the fruits of your labor.

I have watched patients achieve the pinnacle of success only to have a stroke or heart attack remind them that along the way they neglected to give their bodies proper attention. Granted, spastic colon/nervous stomach/IBS is not a life-threatening condition such as a stroke or heart attack, but negligence will result in troublesome symptoms. The stress arising from uncontrolled symptoms of IBS will only compound other medical problems. I have found that the threat of a future disease is less a motivating factor than the immediate benefits many IBS sufferers obtain from dietary changes. This chapter will help you develop a structured approach to eating and meal planning. And once developed, this plan can be continually refined to help you enjoy a full life.

Using a Nutrition Planner

The suggestions in this chapter should steer you onto the right track and motivate you to absorb new information as you expand your knowledge of proper nutrition and diet. Consider using a dietitian as your personal "nutrition planner" during your quest to obtain digestive health. The dietitians I have worked with have been most helpful in assisting my patients identify their specific food intolerances, develop healthful meal plans (which ultimately benefit the entire family), perform dietary analysis to ensure that all nutritional requirements are met (particularly if you are on a restricted diet), and serve as personal tutors, advisers, and sources of encouragement.

It has always struck me as odd that people will spend hundreds of dollars on prepackaged diets for weight reduction, or for body building, and yet be reluctant to invest a fraction of that amount in individualized counseling with a professional dietitian. (And I find it difficult to understand why they think nutrition in a can is more appealing than eating whole foods.)

There are lots of "nutrition experts" out there, and I suggest you shop carefully for your personal nutrition planner. Ask your friends, your doctor, or others whose opinions you value, for their names. Contact them to see if they are willing to meet with you for a get-acquainted visit. At this time, they will most likely outline their approach to proper diet and nutrition. Most dietitians will request that you keep a record of your food intake. This helps them determine your present dietary habits and discover your food preferences. They may also enter this information into a special dietary computer program for a detailed analysis of your intake of fat, carbohydrates, protein, vitamins, and minerals.

The food intake record serves as a base from which the dietitian can make recommendations for dietary modifications. As previously mentioned, these records are also useful in helping to determine food intolerance.

Some dietitians accompany their clients on a grocery store field trip as part of the program. This is a great place both to talk about and learn about food—much better than a classroom. In addition, the clients learn to read package labels. Understanding these labels is a simple task and an essential part of comprehensive nutritional education. Label reading is explored later in this chapter.

There are a multitude of benefits to a well-structured nutritional plan besides the obvious one of lessened digestive symptoms. For many, weight control is a continual concern, and particularly as we age those extra pounds seem to sneak up on us. Eating right can help control weight, and a well-balanced diet will also increase your energy level, enhance your self-image, and even help prevent disease and sickness in the future.

In an earlier chapter, you learned to play detective and identify some foods that are bothersome to you. I hope that your list of food sensitivities is not too long or too restrictive. Ideally, the sufferer will be able to consume, with minimal modification, what everyone else in the family eats. And often, when the family diet is modified to accommodate the sufferer, the changes will ultimately benefit all. Always remember that you can return to your baseline diet as needed when you suffer a flare-up of digestive symptoms.

Visiting a Grocery Store

Living near a grocery store is a mixed blessing. It is certainly convenient when you need to pick up something you forgot or must replenish an item you unexpectedly deplete. However, this convenience makes carefully planned shopping excursions less likely. Many of my patients are from rural eastern Colorado, and I sense that their trips to town for groceries are very well planned. If they happen to omit an item, well, they usually make do. In addition, a last-minute trip to the store for a critical ingredient of your dinner is an added source of stress and a waste of your valuable time.

By now you may begin to sense that the recommendations in this book are all interrelated. Proper meal planning is another way to help reduce stress while following a proper diet, and this combination of proper diet and stress reduction will, in turn, lessen digestive symptoms.

The first step in planning your grocery shopping is to list those items you need. Now, if you are like me, you may need to tie a string around your finger to remember the list. Ideally, you should keep a continual list as you notice you are running out of staples such as milk or bread. Encourage your entire family to use this list, adding those special items they need, or they note are in short supply. Conduct a periodic inventory to identify items not on the list. It is a good idea to maintain a complete list of items you frequently use as a reminder of what to check during your inventory. If you are out of a regularly used item, rather than just low, you may not have a nearly empty container to remind you, but your master list will.

The next step is to prepare a basic menu for the week, or for at least until the next trip to the grocery store. Then add to your list the special ingredients you need for each selected recipe. Now your grocery list should be complete. You may want to arrange the list into various food groups, such as produce, dairy products, and bakery items, to help you save even more time in the store. Saving time in the store will allow you extra time to prepare dinner or simply relax.

Attempt to grocery shop when you are feeling well. The sight and smell of food may make you nauseous or uncomfortable if you must shop while your symptoms are heightened. Avoid shopping when hungry because you may then tend to overbuy. Stick to the list, but take advantage of seasonal availability or "good buys" on items you know you will use. Whenever possible, buy fresh or unsprayed foods; their nutritional value is greater than that of frozen or canned foods. Organic produce is preferable where available.

Try to arrange your grocery trip for a time when the store is not likely to be crowded. This saves additional time, since you will not have to wait in long checkout lines or battle crowded aisles.

How to Read Food Labels

A few years ago, the FDA redesigned food labels to emphasize a diet that is lower in fat, particularly saturated fat, cholesterol, and sodium. Other than vitamin A, vitamin C, calcium, and iron, the old vitamin information is missing. Depending on the product, "Nutrition Facts" on the re-designed food label lays out a "serving size" of so many ounces, wafers, cups, or whatever the appropriate measure is and then tells you how many servings are in the can, bottle, or package. These food labels are representative of the actual serving that people normally eat. The former food labels were very misleading in this regard, often listing one or two crackers as the "serving size."

Calories per serving are listed with the subheading of calories from fat, total fats with a subheading with the percentage that are saturated fat listed in grams and those are related to "percent daily value for a 2000 calorie diet." The same type of listings are made for cholesterol in grams, sodium in milligrams, total carbohydrates in grams (with a subheading for dietary fiber and sugars), and for protein in grams. The "2000 calorie diet" represents a compromise in the "one-size-fits-all" label; 2000 calories may be low for the average male or active person and high for other people who are attempting to lose weight, are smaller or who lead relatively sedentary lives. Moving down the list you will find the percent of required daily values for the four essential nutrients: vitamins A and C, calcium, and iron. You will find the same

Nutrition Facts	
Serving Size 1 oz. (28g/about 12 chips)	
Servings Per Container about 6	

Amount Per Serving	
Calories 120	Calories from Fat 45
	% Daily Value*
Total Fat 5g	8%
Saturated Fat 0g	0%
Cholesterol 0mg	0%
Sodium 10mg	1%
Total Carbohydrates 20g	7%
Dietary Fiber 7g	28%
Sugars 9g	
Protein 0g	

Vitamin A 0%	Vitamin C 10%
Calcium 0%	Iron 2%

*Percent Daily Values are based on a 2,000 calorie diet. Your daily values may be higher or lower depending on your calorie needs:

	Calories:	2,000	2,500
Total Fat	Less than	65g	80g
Sat Fat	Less than	20g	25g
Cholesterol		300mg	300mg
Sodium		2,400mg	2,400mg
Total Carbohydrates		300mg	375mg
Dietary Fiber		25g	30g

listings for fat, cholesterol, sodium, total carbohydrates, and protein as recommended numbers for daily diets of 2000 and 2500 calories per day.

The FDA concludes that the American diet should contain no more than 30 percent fat calories. The average American diet contains 34 to 37

LABELING TERMS

The following is a list of terms and definitions imposed by federal regulation to describe various food products. This list may be helpful as you attempt to decrease your intake of fat, sodium, or calories:

U.S.

Extra Lean	Less than 5 percent fat.
Lean or Low Fat	Less than 10 percent fat.
Lite, Leaner, or Lower Fat	At least 25 percent less fat than similar products.
Sodium Free	Fewer than 5 mg per serving.
Very Low Sodium	Fewer than 35 mg per serving.
Low Sodium	Fewer than 140 mg per serving.
Reduced Sodium	At least a 75 percent reduction compared with the usual content of the food.
Unsalted	No salt added during processing.
Low Calorie	No more than 40 calories per serving, or no more than 0.4 calories per gram.
Reduced Calorie	Minimum of 1/3 fewer calories compared with usual product.

Canada

Fat Free	Less than 0.1 g fat per 100 g serving.
Low Fat or Light	Less than 3 g fat per serving.
Reduced in Fat	More than a 25 percent reduction compared with similar products.
Salt Free	Less than 5 mg per 100 g serving.
Low Sodium, Low in Sodium, or Light in Salt	Less than 40 mg sodium per 100 g serving (50 mg sodium/100 g for cheddar cheese, and 80 mg for meat, poultry, and fish). At least a 50 percent reduction in sodium.
No Salt Added or Unsalted	No sodium added, and no ingredient contributes a significant amount of sodium.
Reduced Sodium	At least a 25 percent reduction in salt.
Low Calorie, Light in Calories, or Low in Energy	A 50 percent reduction in calories. No more than 15 calories per average serving, and 30 calories per reasonable daily intake.
Reduced in Calories, Lower in Calories	More than 25 percent reduction in energy.
Calorie Reduced, Light in Calories	A 50 percent reduction compared with the usual content of the food.

percent fat. Many experts would contend that an ideal diet would contain no more than 10 to 20 percent fat. The FDA's new labeling rules also contain definitions for such terms as light, low fat, and less or reduced fat.

There are a few little known facts about the listing of ingredients in labels. One is that ingredients are listed in the order of their volume. In other words, if flour is the main ingredient, it will be listed first, and so on. Another little known fact is that MSG is often represented in other terms, such as hydrolyzed protein and glutamic acid. Often, incidental additives used in processing that are considered insignificant and without a technical or functional effect on the processed food are not listed on labels. (See Chapter 5 for a list of food additives to avoid.)

Foods advertised for their nutritional properties, such as "low-fat" or "low-calorie" products, and foods that have been enriched or fortified, such as breakfast cereals, are required by law to have nutritional labels. Other products may voluntarily carry nutritional information on their labels. In both cases, the label must list the total number of calories and the number of grams of protein, carbohydrate, and fat per serving.

Nutrition labels in the United States must also include the percentage of the U.S. Recommended Daily Allowances (U.S. RDA) for eight nutrients: protein, calcium, iron, vitamin A, vitamin C, thiamine, riboflavin, and niacin. A listing of other nutrients, such as vitamin D, may be included but is not required. In Canada, nutrient labels are not mandatory, but where they are used, fat, protein, energy, and carbohydrate levels must be listed. However, manufacturers are not required to state levels of vitamins or mineral nutrients, such as iron or zinc.

TIPS ABOUT CALCULATING FAT CALORIES

There are approximately nine calories in every gram of fat, and four calories per gram of carbohydrate or protein. Remember this relationship and you can easily calculate the percentage of fat calories contained within a product. For example, a cup of whole milk contains 150 calories with eight grams of protein; 11 grams of carbohydrates; and eight grams of fat.

By multiplying grams of fat by calories per gram (8 grams x 9 calories per gram), we get 72 calories; almost half of the 150 total calories in a cup of whole milk is derived from fat. This means a cup of skim milk, which contains no fat, has approximately 78 calories (150 − 72). You can see the tremendous decrease in calories, particularly fat calories, you achieve by switching from whole milk (approximately 3.5 percent milk fat) to skim milk.

Preparing a Weekly Menu

Ideally, food preparation begins shortly after your return from shopping. Resealable plastic bags, airtight plastic containers, and recycled glass jars are an invaluable aid for keeping foods fresh and saving leftovers. You may wish to rinse and chop vegetables at this time and store them for later use. Lettuce that is washed, drained, and placed in an airtight container will last longer and is ready for use at any time. If simply tossed into the refrigerator, lettuce—and other vegetables—will often wilt within a few days. The fact is, you are much more likely to eat salads and fresh vegetables if they are already washed and ready for consumption.

This is also a good time to skin and debone chicken or to filet fish for later use. This will save you time later on, since much of the preliminary work for using these ingredients in a meal will already have been done. Some experts suggest that when you prepare foods in advance, they lose nutrients and freshness. I believe that if this preparation is carried out properly, the loss—if any—will be minimal. The following suggestions will help you enjoy tasty, home-cooked, nutritious meals with a minimum of stress.

Use discarded leafy tops of vegetables and chicken bones for making stock. The more fresh foods you prepare from scratch, the less likely you are to encounter the troublesome ingredients found in prepackaged food.

It is more efficient and economical to prepare larger quantities of certain foods—which you can easily refrigerate or freeze for later use—than to prepare each meal from scratch. This way, you have homemade "TV dinners" whenever you lack the time or desire to cook. Some items, such as soups, stews, spaghetti sauce, and casseroles, actually seem to taste better as leftovers. If you are not sure whether you will be using an item within a few days, store it in the freezer rather than allowing it to deteriorate in the refrigerator. Label all containers and include the date. Always throw out any food that may have spoiled. Do not feed it to the dog unless you are prepared to eat it yourself. (Why make Fido sick?)

A New Way of Reducing Stress

Bret was a single executive who hated to cook. He actually felt uncomfortable in the kitchen, and the sum total of his experience in the culinary arts consisted of proficient use of the microwave and toaster. His specialty was microwave popcorn. He knew the precise temperature setting and timing to make a perfect batch.

As Bret advanced within the corporate structure, his stress level increased, and it was at this time that he was referred to me. After reviewing his food intake record, I realized that his diet was a major contributor to his symptoms. But I also felt certain he would be unable to change his dietary habits without some help. Fortunately, the dietitian recommended to him worked with a cook who would not only grocery shop for clients but would actually prepare meals in the home for future consumption.

At first, Bret was not receptive to the idea of having a personal cook twice weekly; he thought it would be far too costly. He agreed, however, to try it briefly, and the result was a dramatic improvement in his symptoms. He remarked, during a later visit with me, that he felt he was actually saving money because he was brown-bagging it at lunch time and eating out less. His personalized lunches and dinners were comparable in cost to the frozen dinners he had been buying at the store. Brown-bagging is a sensible, cost-efficient way to control the quantity and content of the food you eat while enjoying home-cooked meals when you are out.

Americans consume more than one-third of their meals outside the home. Given this information, it is encouraging that more restaurants are developing health-conscious menu items. In the next section, there are some preventive health hints for dining away from home.

Eating Outside the Home

Diane called our office one morning seeking advice for intense abdominal cramps and diarrhea. I had not spoken to her in some months, and asked what she thought had triggered this latest episode. Apparently, she had attended a dinner party at a friend's home the previous evening. She was famished when she arrived because she had skipped lunch to run errands and to take one of her children to a doctor. When the host offered wine with cheese and crackers as starters, she could not resist. The appetizer served only to whet her appetite, and when the home-made lasagna arrived, she attacked her plate.

Diane knew she had a low tolerance for lactose-containing foods; had she remembered her lactase enzyme supplements, perhaps she might not have been in her present predicament. She also recalled, the next day, that alcohol, particularly wine, had caused problems in the past. Although she had declined at first, her host insisted she try "a taste." He was right; the wine hit the spot, and after the first glass, she found it even more difficult to decline a refill.

This story suggests several important points. First, you should give as much thought and preparation to the meals you will eat out as to those you eat at home. Depending on the situation, ask what will be served. Tell the host or hostess ahead of time that you have a digestive disorder (you need not go into any more detail) and that your doctor has suggested you restrict consumption of certain foods. In most instances, your hosts will be able to modify your serving (for example, giving you less gravy, sauce, or cheese) or provide a suitable alternative. At least they will be less likely to insist that you try the wine, rich desserts, or espresso if they know ahead of time that you must exercise dietary discretion. You will end up feeling better and also be more convincing if, for example, you compliment the chef but actually eat only half a portion.

In addition, Diane could have saved herself a lot of discomfort had she remembered her lactase enzyme supplements.

She broke another important rule by arriving at the dinner party hungry. That is not to say she should have eaten a complete meal just before leaving; however, she would have been less inclined to overindulge had she not skipped lunch, or had she eaten a light snack before leaving home. I cannot overemphasize the importance of frequent small meals to help control digestive symptoms.

Alcohol, particularly on an empty stomach, can cause havoc in the digestive tract of an IBS sufferer. It is always a good idea, whether or not you have IBS, to eat a light meal or snack before a cocktail party. This is especially true if you plan to consume alcohol. You will find the alcohol less bothersome, and you will be less likely to overeat. The combination of alcohol and rich hors d'oeuvres does not constitute an ideal meal, and yet if you do not eat something ahead of time, it could very well be your meal for the evening.

Finally, as difficult as it may be at times, be assertive. If you accept and eat a restricted food, you are the one who will pay later. I realize that this will often tax your willpower to the limit, especially when what is offered looks and smells really delicious. You do not want to offend the hostess, and she really has persisted in her request that you "at least try it." As one patient remarked to me, "I get in these situations where my taste buds out-vote my stomach."

Dining in a restaurant can still be a pleasurable experience, although I do encounter patients who worry about eating out because "I never know if or how I will react to the food." In contrast to a dinner party, you do have a little more choice when you are eating out. Seek out restaurants that offer healthful dishes. Unfortunately, although there are no entrees prepared especially with the IBS sufferer in mind, many report that they find "heart-smart," low-cholesterol, low-sodium dishes quite palatable and without negative reactions. These dishes are generally lighter, and the decreased fat content is less likely to cause problems. Do not be afraid to inquire about the use of additives. For example, ask about the use of MSG, particularly if you are planning to dine in an oriental restaurant. Often, it can be omitted on request.

Avoid fried foods. Request that salad dressings, gravies, and sauces be served on the side. This allows you to control the amount you use, and you may find the dishes delicious without these accompaniments. You do not need the extra calories anyway. Since sweets are a common trigger, do not order dessert until after a meal. You may find you have had enough without one. If you really crave something sweet, order some fresh fruit, or share a dessert with someone else.

Meals while Traveling

Many experienced travelers are aware that airlines will provide special meals at no extra cost and that the meal service is not a take-it-or-leave-it proposition. But you must plan ahead and notify the airline at least 24 hours in advance (or tell your travel agent when purchasing the tickets), and request one of their listed special meals. The selections are somewhat limited, but they include a low-calorie, a low-fat, a low-sodium, and a vegetarian meal. These alternatives, although still airline food, are lighter and usually easier to digest than the standard meal.

At your hotel, take advantage of room service if it is provided. In some of the nicer hotels, this is a relaxing way to enjoy an elegant meal in the privacy of your room. And if you can, choose a hotel with exercise facilities to maintain your regular exercise program.

Travel across time zones can often result in jet lag. Rapid transit through time belts, particularly international travel, may lead to fatigue, headaches, and mental clouding. Psychological adjustments may occur quickly, but your physiological functions, such as digestion, kidney performance, hormonal regulation, and the sleep/wake cycle, may take longer to conform to the new schedule. This change is often coupled with a change in diet as you encounter rich, unfamiliar foods during travel. If you are not careful, this may throw your bowels into rebellion. Attempt to stick with your diet and with familiar foods as much as possible when on the road. Take along some "safe" snacks and fiber supplements to use as needed to regularize bowel movements.

If possible, plan to arrive at your destination a day early to allow some time for rest and to begin the adjustment process. You may begin preparation for rhythm disturbances in advance by retiring one hour earlier for each hour to be lost going east, or one hour later for each hour to be gained when traveling west.

 ON AIRLINE TRAVEL

Place an emergency provisions kit in your carry-on luggage, including:

- Herbal tea, individual serving-size boxes of fiber-rich cereal, healthful snacks, lactase enzyme supplements, fiber supplements, and prescribed medications.
- Eat a light meal before departure and avoid gas-producing foods.
- Wear loose-fitting, comfortable clothing.
- Avoid alcohol before and during the flight.

CHAPTER 8

Stress and the Intestinal Tract

in collaboration with Jack Martin, Ph.D.

ALL OF US at some time experience emotions that lead to physiological responses. Blushing in response to an embarrassing situation is a classic example. Have you ever had butterflies in the stomach, or even nervous diarrhea, before giving a speech? The stress of public speaking can cause your palms to sweat, your heart to race, and your knees to turn to noodles. If some people had to give a eulogy at a funeral, they would probably rather be in the coffin!

It is difficult to give an all-inclusive definition of stress, because the word itself has developed many different connotations. Quite simply, stress may be any stimulus that requires adaptation or change. As things are constantly changing in life, the way you react physically and emotionally to change determines how much distress you experience.

Another definition of stress is pressure or strain. The Canadian researcher Hans Selye was one of the first to study stress in the human body. He defined stress as a physical, chemical, or emotional development that causes strain and can lead to physical illness. He described three stages of the stress response:

- In the first stage, alarm, the body recognizes the stress and prepares for action, either to fight or escape. The sympathetic branch of the autonomic nervous system increases the heart and respiratory rate, and increases blood flow to muscles. The endocrine glands release hormones that elevate blood sugar, increase perspiration, dilate the pupils, and slow the digestion.

- In the second stage, resistance, the body repairs any damage caused by the alarm reaction. If the stress continues, the body remains alert and cannot repair the damage.
- As resistance continues, the third stage, exhaustion, sets in, and a stress-related disorder can result. Prolonged exposure to stress depletes the body's energy supplies and can even lead to death.

In recent times, the stress response has been described as the "fight/flight" response. This term is used to describe a process that occurs often unconsciously whenever the brain perceives a threat. When this happens, the body first tries to protect the vital organs, which include the brain, heart, and lungs. Most other parts of the body receive secondary consideration in the fight/flight response. For example, digestion is not considered to be essential to fighting or fleeing.

To understand this unconscious response to perceived threats, consider how we have evolved. Only a few centuries ago, humankind lived in a hostile environment and threats to the body were mostly physical in nature. So over time, we have become programmed to either fight the threat or flee from it—hence the term "fight/flight" response. Today in our technologically developed world, most threats are much less physical and much more emotional in nature. But the body has been programmed to regard threats as physical. Consequently, even a look of displeasure on another person's face can be experienced by the body as if a wild animal is preparing to attack.

To prepare for a threat, either by fighting it or running from it, the body arouses itself to its maximum potential. The heart rate, blood pressure, and temperature increase. Blood flow also changes. When the body is relaxed and not threatened, blood flow is equally distributed throughout the body, with all areas experiencing an equal amount of warmth. When the perception of threat occurs, however, blood tends to move out of the arms and legs, often resulting in a drop in temperature in the hands and feet. This process is accomplished by the constriction of tiny muscles inside the arteries and blood vessels of the arms and legs. Having "cold feet" is an apt description of what happens to us when we feel threatened.

A paradoxical response of the body to threat is that our hands and feet might also sweat. Because the body is preparing itself to either fight or flee, it assumes that it will need to be cooled. The body's natural way of cooling itself is by sweating. The sweating is intended to reduce the heat that will result from fighting or fleeing. Skin moisture is another sign that the body is engaged in a fight/flight response.

The reduction of blood flow to the extremities is also accompanied by the dilation of arteries and blood vessels in the chest and brain area where the vital organs are located. Consequently, a warming of the chest and brain area results, and the skin covering these parts can become red. Headaches can also result as blood flow and subsequent pressure to the brain increases.

At the same time, the arteries and blood vessels in the digestive area constrict because digestion is not crucial for fighting or fleeing from a threat. This reduction of blood flow can precipitate a variety of gastrointestinal problems, including IBS. Frequent complaints of digestive problems are another sign of the fight/flight response.

The stress response also changes our breathing patterns. When the brain perceives a threat, breathing becomes short and shallow. For example, when some people are startled, they immediately gasp for air. This change in breathing pattern to short and shallow can result in too much carbon dioxide in the brain, which triggers the fight/flight response.

Another part of the fight/flight response involves muscle tension. When a threat is perceived, muscles immediately begin to tighten. If the perception of threat continues, chronic muscle tension results, which can become chronic muscle pain.

TIPS ABOUT STRESS AND BREATHING PATTERNS

Adequate respiration is crucial to managing stress. Biofeedback is one stress management technique that allows individuals to observe their breathing patterns and change them, often resulting in reduction of IBS symptoms.

It is important to remember that often what causes the fight/flight response is not what happens to us, but rather our perception of what happens to us. In North America, we are bombarded by media (news, advertising, and entertainment) that often portrays many situations as threatening. As a result, many of us habitually respond to circumstances with the fight/flight response. Let's look at the physiological response to a perceived threat that can occur in a common, real-life setting.

Imagine you have just finished your evening meal and decide to take a relaxing stroll around the neighborhood. Although it is already dark, you are unconcerned because your neighborhood is considered relatively safe. Strolling in a leisurely fashion past a row of bushes, you note they have not been trimmed lately and resolve to bring up this fact at the next neighborhood meeting. Suddenly you hear a rustling among the leaves. A large figure looms out of the darkness holding a long shiny object. You are overcome with fear, sensing imminent danger.

Without thinking about it, your sympathetic nervous system is stimulated to prepare you for this threat. Your pupils dilate, you breathe faster, begin salivating (to keep your windpipe from drying out while breathing), and your pulse quickens. Your muscles tense as they receive increased blood flow, which has been shifted away from your digestive organs, and your adrenal and thyroid glands increase their secretion of stored hormones.

Thoughts race through your mind as you contemplate your options: should I run, or should I stand my ground and use the self-defense techniques I learned in tae kwon do last summer?

You realize your throat is so tight you could not yell for help if you wanted to. Then, as the figure moves into full view in the light afforded by a street lamp, you recognize your neighbor carrying a pair of hedge clippers. "Nice evening for a walk, isn't it?" he declares. "I simply can't seem to find time to trim these hedges during the day, so I thought I'd work on them tonight."

A few moments later you continue your walk. Your sympathetic nervous system begins to wind down, and your parasympathetic system decreases your heart and respiration rate and increases blood flow to your digestive system so that you can relax and digest your dinner.

Chronic Stress

Is all stress bad? No. Actually, under appropriate circumstances, so-called positive stress stimulates creativity, facilitates change, and may help you reach peak efficiency. Many people work quite well under pressure and are able to sit back and relax after meeting the challenge. This relaxation response allows them to accumulate the physical and emotional reserves needed to meet the next task. Stress becomes negative when you remain geared up, and are unable to relax after the challenge. You become like the crew of a warship that remains ready at all battle stations long after the threat is over. This continual state of arousal sets up a perpetual energy-draining cycle, which causes your health and well-being to suffer.

The American Digestive Disease Society considers stress a disease. In fact, this may be the best way to view chronic stress. When life's daily stresses result in chronic distress, it is usually the result of a prolonged arousal of the sympathetic branch of the autonomic system. This prolonged arousal shows itself in different ways in different people: tension headaches, chest discomfort, fatigue, muscle aches, susceptibility to infection, and IBS. Some IBS sufferers attribute stress to be the primary cause of their symptoms. Others cannot accept stress as a possible contributing factor to their symptoms because they cannot identify the stresses in their lives.

You may feel that you have no stresses in your life, that you have a nice family, a good job, and so on. However, for many, chronic stress is an insidious, pervasive problem. It may not be the result of readily identifiable life events, such as divorce or the death of a loved one. Indeed, untreated symptoms of an illness such as IBS may be a source of continued stress perpetuating the stress-illness-stress cycle. Your IBS symptoms can also produce stress in your relationships. In a recent study, 71 percent of those with IBS said their significant relationships had been disrupted by the disorder (refer to Chapter 11 for more information regarding IBS and relationships). Uncontrolled symptoms can interfere with sexual activity, and result in marital discord. The resultant heightened tensions may, in turn, worsen IBS symptoms, and so on.

This is not to say that stress is always the root of IBS symptoms. But to the extent that you learn to recognize the symptoms of stress, and learn to deal effectively with them, you will be able to exert more control in your life and avoid or eliminate chronic stress.

Tracking Stress

We all have various stresses in our lives, and how we perceive stress and deal with it determines how much distress we experience. The first step in learning to manage stress is to identify the stresses in your life. Remember that a situation that is perceived as a threat will lead to the stress response. And be aware that a stressful event for one person may not cause much stress in another. Sometimes it may be difficult to pinpoint the most significant stresses in your life, such as subconscious worries, marital conflicts, financial pressures, or lack of self-confidence.

If you are prone to stress, closely examine your attitudes. Do you make unrealistic demands on yourself? Do you always attempt to control every situation? Do you feel unfulfilled if all of your goals are not met? How you relate to the people and events in your life may be a source of chronic stress, if these relationships are not addressed and dealt with appropriately.

Keeping a stress diary is an effective method of tracking stress. You can expand the diet diary illustrated in Chapter 5 and add more items to note about stress. You can begin by reviewing the stresses listed in this chapter, and note any of them that you are experiencing. Note the date and degree of stress on a scale of one to five, with five being "most stressful." If the stress is ongoing, note that as well, along with its cause. Also include how you feel about the stress and whether it is positive, negative, neutral, or a combination of these.

After identifying the stresses, you must learn to "listen to your body" for related symptoms: headaches, tension, fatigue, or disordered defecation patterns. List the IBS symptoms that occur with the stresses. Biofeedback is another way to connect stresses to symptoms. See pages 95–96 to find out how biofeedback training can help with IBS.

Keep your stress diary for a period of two weeks. Then take time to review it and discuss the findings with your doctor. He or she may help you develop stress management strategies, or refer you to a counselor to identify underlying causes of stress that you cannot discover by yourself.

Stress Management

As earlier mentioned, the same stress that affects one individual minimally may affect another individual with much greater intensity. You may have planned and shopped ahead for Christmas, as you look forward to being with family and friends. Conversely, you may be one who has to rush around at the last minute to find the "perfect" gift for everyone on your holiday list. An individual's personality often dictates whether or not a given degree of stress results in distress.

The classic Type A perfectionist personalities place undue stress on their systems by making unrealistic demands of themselves. They are often disappointed and depressed when they do not achieve their unrealistic goals. (See Chapter 11 for a thorough discussion of how perfectionism results in IBS symptoms and how it can be treated.) Stress-prone individuals often feel that they are victims of circumstances with no control over their lives or environments—they tend to approach life with a certain degree of negativity and defensiveness.

Although we cannot control all of the events in our lives that cause stress, most of us have much more control than we realize. We can learn to focus our energies appropriately and achieve balance and harmony. We also can avoid stressful situations whenever possible. For example, if you hate getting caught in traffic, try leaving for work a little earlier, when the streets are less crowded.

Often, learning to manage your time more effectively is an excellent way to reduce chronic stress. You may find you are wasting a lot of your time and energy running around needlessly working on projects that should be given a much lower priority. I strongly recommend the book

Time Power by Charles R. Hobbs, or his cassette series, *Your Time and Your Life*. Hobbs says that "time management is the act of controlling events" so that you achieve "balance, harmony and appropriateness among the events in your life."

Here is an example of how time management relieved a working mother's IBS symptoms. Barbara, a 33-year-old housewife and book-keeper, worked outside the home from 9:00 a.m. to 3:00 p.m., four days a week, doing bookkeeping for a dentist. She complained mainly of constipation and intermittent abdominal cramps. A social history revealed that she was, in every way, a Supermom, Superwife, and Superemployee. But Barbara never took time for herself. She related: "I don't even have time to go to the bathroom."

The prescription for Barbara was to schedule time during the week for herself. At first, she expressed guilt about taking this time. But it was pointed out to her that she couldn't continue her present course because it was damaging her health. She was doing great things for her children, her husband, and her employer, but she was neglecting to care for herself with the same diligence.

Barbara's husband wholeheartedly agreed with the prescription. He described his wife as a person who "could never say no." He also commented that, financially speaking, she had no need to work outside the home as much as she did; the young dentist she worked for had gradually asked her to increase her hours as his practice grew.

Barbara is now job sharing, cutting back to two days a week. She rises a little earlier each morning before the children and uses this time to read, relax, and plan her day. On her last office visit, she proudly announced: "My stomach no longer bothers me, and our family life is as good as it ever was." She and her husband now plan at least one night a week to enjoy "dates" together.

Relaxation Techniques for Stress

For stressful situations that are unavoidable, there are relaxation techniques that have proved very successful. Stress management consists of first identifying the things in your life that cause you to feel stress. Second, you learn to focus on how you feel under stress. Finally, when you begin to feel stress in the form of distress, you need to be able to relax. When you relax, you will notice a decrease in muscular tension, a slowing of your heart rate, slowing of your respiration rate, and facilitation of the digestive process.

You may already use some relaxation techniques from time to time, such as taking a warm bath, listening to music, working in the garden, going for a walk, or reading a good book. However, there are other, more specific relaxation techniques that can be learned and practiced to become an integral part of your daily life. In this way, you can use daily stress reduction as a means of achieving a higher level of health.

As discussed earlier, rapid breathing is a response to stress. In contrast, breathing slowly and deeply is an obvious way to neutralize stress. This basic relaxation technique can be performed anywhere and at

TIPS ON STRESS MANAGEMENT

Your stress management program must be comprehensive to significantly improve your health. Make sure you include all of the following:
• Adequate exercise
• Proper nutrition
• Adequate relaxation and play activities
• Adequate sleep
• Meaningful work
• Quiet, contemplation, and meditation
• Receiving and giving love
• Perceiving life events and relationships with a positive outlook

any time. It is a good idea to practice deep breathing for a few minutes several times during the day, but particularly if you begin to feel tense.

Here's how: Place your hands over your abdomen and feel your stomach expand. Inhale slowly and deeply through your nose. Hold your breath for a second or two, then very slowly exhale through your mouth. Repeat this cycle several times until you feel at ease. While continuing to breathe in this conscious manner, listen to a relaxation tape with soothing words and music, such as the one I have produced for my IBS patients, *Stress and IBS*. (See Appendix 5, "Resources," for details on how to order this tape.)

Another useful relaxation technique involves visual imagery, which is similar to daydreaming. It is best performed while sitting upright in a comfortable chair. Assume a relaxed position, then let your mind take you on a mental vacation. For example, you are lying on a beach and there is beautiful sunshine. You feel the warm rays on your skin, and a cool, gentle breeze. With each breath, your body is invigorated by the clean, fresh air. You hear waves splashing against the shore and sea gulls calling in the distance.

With practice, you can learn to give yourself well-deserved mental vacations with relative ease. One word of caution: Never practice your relaxation techniques in a situation requiring you to be fully alert, such as while driving or reading this book!

Progressive muscle relaxation is another easily learned relaxation technique. It is most helpful for those who report feeling tense. This technique is best performed in a quiet environment, either sitting or lying down. The basic procedure takes about 15 minutes and consists of alternately contracting and relaxing various muscle groups. In this way, you learn to distinguish between control and relaxation. Begin by contracting the muscles around the eyes, as you would if you were squinting in a sand storm. Hold the tension a few seconds, then relax. Repeat the cycle three times before moving to another group of muscles. By the time you have moved from head to toe, your muscles should be warm and relaxed. Yoga and various martial arts, such as tai chi, combine muscular activity and mental relaxation; as one yoga instructor explained, "It's like meditation in motion."

Exercise is another excellent means of reducing stress and tension, and physically fit people tend to handle stress more easily than unfit people. The important role of exercise is discussed in Chapter 10, "The Importance of Proper Exercise."

If you lack self-confidence or find it difficult to be assertive, consider taking a self-help course to learn better communication skills. For stressful situations that are unavoidable, there are many other relaxation techniques that have proved very successful.

BIOFEEDBACK TRAINING
An Effective Treatment for Stress and IBS

BIOFEEDBACK TRAINING is an effective means of stress management by gaining control of the body using the mind. These techniques are also very useful in treating many health problems, including IBS. In fact, research by the National Institutes of Health has shown that biofeedback can reduce symptoms of bowel disorders by 75 to 80 percent.

Biofeedback uses a computer to monitor bodily functions, such as heart rate, muscle tension, respiration patterns, skin moisture, hand and foot temperature, and brain wave activity. The computer is connected to the body in several different ways. For example, to discover muscle tension, small electrodes are placed on muscle sites to measure the amount of electricity sent by the brain. Other electrodes are attached to the skin to measure skin moisture, indicating whether the body is in a fight/flight response. A small thermometer is attached to the skin to measure skin temperature, an indirect measure of blood flow and the amount of stress in the cardiovascular system. Electrodes can also be attached to the scalp area; this type of feedback is called neurotherapy, and allows an individual to observe and modify brainwave activity.

The feedback that comes from the attached sensors is displayed in graphs, charts, pictures of various types, and auditory signals. By observing this feedback while using stress management techniques, you know immediately whether or not the techniques are effective. For example, you can observe how your breathing patterns are bringing oxygen into the bloodstream. Biofeedback respiration training involves attaching a Velcro belt to the waist area to measure the expansion of the diaphragm area. First you observe the computer feedback of the effects of your normal breathing pattern. (It is normal to breathe in for about two seconds and breathe out for about two seconds.) Then you consciously change your breathing pattern to breathe in for approximately four seconds and breathe out for four seconds, with a one-second pause between the two. During this exercise, you observe immediate feedback from the computer regarding various physiological measurements that indicate a heightened state of relaxation.

With training, you can often learn how to alter heart rate, blood pressure, blood flow, muscle tension, chronic pain due to muscle tension and stress, skin moisture, headaches, and gastrointestinal problems. In many cases, it is necessary to examine how you perceive your circumstances and health problems. Remember—most stress comes from the perception of threat, so if we can change the way we look at life, we may also be able to change the way we react to it. Let's look at how biofeedback helped a person with IBS improve her health and marriage.

Grace was in her early 70s and had been suffering from IBS for a number of years. She was referred by her internist for biofeedback training when he suspected a link between stress and IBS. An initial consultation revealed that Grace suffered from a great deal of emotional tension at home. She felt her husband was overbearing and controlling. She wanted to travel but her husband rarely wanted to leave home, which frustrated and angered her. Instead of sharing her feelings, she buried them and became increasingly angry. Whenever his behavior angered her, IBS symptoms erupted. Truly, her IBS was both a barometer and a means of expressing her feelings.

We initiated biofeedback to first observe the physical symptoms that contributed to IBS. We noticed that her hand temperature was in the low 70-degree range. In addition, the muscle tension in her shoulder area was elevated. We worked with changing her breathing patterns by using a respiration belt to measure the amount of expansion in the diaphragm area. By taking in more oxygen into the blood stream, Grace learned how to relax. Increased blood flow and oxygen to the gastrointestinal tract also improved her digestion and elimination processes.

Grace also began to learn more about her emotions and improve her communication skills. She kept a daily journal, noting her emotional states when her IBS symptoms occurred. She noticed that symptoms were worse when she was upset with either her husband, close friends, or herself. In consultation, I asked her to fully describe why she was upset, and we discussed alternative ways of dealing with her emotions. I encouraged her to be more open with her feelings, first by writing about them and then by sharing them with her husband and friends in a respectful way. Over the course of time, we created effective strategies for dealing with her anger. To her surprise, Grace's husband was not as hostile toward her openness as she had feared. In fact, he began to respect her more.

Within eight weeks of beginning biofeedback and stress management training, Grace was IBS-symptom free. Not only had she improved her marriage, but she had also gained mastery of her body and emotions. In subsequent weeks, whenever IBS symptoms appeared, she was able to identify the underlying frustration or anger and quickly deal with it by practicing biofeedback techniques and communication skills.

by Dr. Jack Martin

CHAPTER 9

Understanding the Psychophysiology of IBS

by Paul B. Donovan, Ph.D.

B Y THIS CHAPTER, you probably have a good understanding of the connection between stress, diet, and IBS symptoms. Current research in the psychobiology of IBS reveals even more connections to symptoms—the underlying physiology, events in our daily lives, and the psychophysiological processes by which these events become IBS triggers. For example, we now know that many IBS sufferers have a magnified neurological sensitivity to bowel sensations, so that it only takes a little stress to create an intense sensation.

In my practice as a psychophysiologist and director of an IBS clinic in Santa Fe, New Mexico, I use this research in developing a self-help treatment plan for each individual. The treatment plan incorporates cognitive behavioral therapy—a four-step method of information control, cognitive control, behavioral control, and autonomic control. The word "control" is important because so many IBS sufferers report a loss of control, not only with rectal urgency (which results in agoraphobia, a fear of being in open or public places) but also a loss of control in their whole lives.

Information control aims at clarifying some of the myths and misinformation surrounding IBS. I use dozens of illustrations of different kinds to explain the physiology and psychophysiology of IBS, which provide people with a unifying explanation for what is happening to their bodies.

THE AUTONOMIC TRIAD

**When the autonomic nervous system is on "overdrive,"
multiple syndromes result.**

THYROID ⟶
HYPOGLYCEMIA ⟶
DIABETES ⟶

IBS
IRRITABLE BOWEL
SYNDROME
(gastrointestinal system)

FMS
FIBROMYALGIA
SYNDROME
(musculoskeletal system)

CFIDS
CHRONIC FATIGUE IMMUNO-
DEFICIENCY SYNDROME
(auto-immune system)

diarrhea/constipation

muscle aches
and pains

chronic colds,
sore throat, fatigue
(post-viral recovery)

The same person may have elements of all three of these syndromes,
and the predominant syndrome may shift over time.

© Copyright 2001 Paul Donovan, Ph. D.

The autonomic nervous system (and associated neuroendocrine system) is the body's "engine" that accelerates or brakes its functioning to respond to outer events. The significance of these events is "filtered" by the conscious mind. For example, a cocktail party may be a source of fun and relaxation for one person, but may fill another with foreboding, resentment, and the fear of social scrutiny and embarrassment. In addition, thyroid imbalances, hypoglycemia, diabetes, and other medical disorders may also disturb the functioning of the autonomic-enteric nervous system.

The cognitive-behavioral components identify automatic patterns of thinking and reacting (such as perfectionism), which are self-defeating for the individual. This method is best done by a health psychologist who is familiar with the psychophysiology of functional gastrointestinal disorders.

Autonomic control seeks to lower the level at which the autonomic-enteric nervous system is "turned on," which, in the case of IBS sufferers, is often on "overdrive" like a car engine revving too fast. (This condition is also called autonomic hyperactivity or dysautonomia.) The autonomic nervous system responds to the mind's perceptions of the external world and regulates the internal organs to match those perceptions of external demands, slowing down or speeding up as required, changing blood flow (vasoconstriction or vasodilation) and muscle tension (both the internal smooth muscle of the colon and esophagus as well as the external striated muscle). It's easy to see then, why headaches, fibromyalgia, and chronic fatigue (the so-called autonomic triad) are often associated with IBS.

Various medications can be used to stabilize autonomic hyperactivity and improve IBS symptoms. However, in the 1930s, Harvard physician and physiologist Edmund Jacobson developed a means of autonomic control using a skill instead of a pill. This is called neuromuscular retraining and is based on the principle that autonomic elevation always increases muscle tension. Jacobson realized this neurological connection and wondered whether the reverse applies, so that lowering muscle tension would lower the level of autonomic functioning. He developed a means of doing this, wrote a best-selling book on his wonderful discovery, *You Must Relax* (McGraw-Hill, 1934), and founded the modern relaxation movement.

How Automatic Patterns Affect the Autonomic System

Most people with IBS have self-defeating patterns of thinking and behaving which reinforce themselves and become automatic responses. If IBS sufferers could have changed these patterns, they would have already done so and their condition may not have become chronic.

AUTONOMIC PATHWAYS

When there is a chronic arousal of the autonomic nervous system, different people develop symptoms in different organs.

- hypertension
- palpitations (arrhythmias)
- vasoconstriction (tingling, numbness or coldness)
- migraine
- skin rash (urticaria)

- colds (reduced antibodies)
- sinus

- TMJ
- fibromyalgia
- tension headache
- lower back pain

CHRONIC AUTONOMIC AROUSAL

- functional dyspepsia
- IBS
- oesophageal spasm
- non-cardiac chest pain ("cardiac neurosis")
- nausea

- hyperventilation syndrome
- panic disorder

A hyperactive autonomic nervous system can also be a genetic inheritance, however. People with such a disposition are very sensitive to what is happening around them; they tend to take on more tasks than they can handle and then collapse. A hyperactive autonomic nervous system can also result from life experiences: a childhood or adolescent experience of sexual or physical abuse or a family culture of constant conflict can produce a hypothalamic-pituitary-adrenal imbalance (the "trigger mechanism" for autonomic regulation), resulting in IBS. Later life experiences, such as an automobile accident or a lengthy viral illness, combined with a "highly strung" autonomic-endocrine system, can result in post-traumatic, chronic symptoms such as IBS. Often it's not the trauma itself, but the profound loss of personal control and sense of powerlessness that plunges the autonomic system into irregularity. In addition, thyroid or cholesterol abnormalities, menses or menopause in women, diabetes or hypoglycemia can also affect the autonomic nervous system due to endocrine changes that "shock" the system.

Whatever the causes, when self-defeating patterns of thinking and feeling are present with problems of anxiety or depression, the body habitually responds to circumstances with alarm, fear, or overload. Over time, this alarm response alters the automatic functioning of the smooth muscle surrounding the colon. At this stage, not only does the autonomic nervous system become disordered, so too does the associated enteric nervous system—the so-called gut-brain or the body's second brain that regulates neurological signals sent to the colonic smooth muscle.

Understanding how the smooth muscle around the colon functions can help you to gain more control of how your body reacts to your own thoughts, feelings, and daily circumstances. The autonomic nervous system activates or relaxes organs such as the heart, lungs, and gastrointestinal tract according to your perception of circumstances. For example, if you have a "nervous stomach" that reacts to stress, your body may use the existing psychophysiological "pathway" of the intestinal tract to provide a distraction for disturbing thoughts. You then become preoc-

THE BIOPSYCHOSOCIAL CYCLE OF IBS

SOCIAL-
Lifestyle Events
- Loss of parent
- Behavior problems with children
- Conflict with spouse
- Work demands/ personality conflicts
- Fear of losing job

PSYCHO-
Processing of Events by the Brain
- Perceptual distortion
- Hypervigilance
- Rumination
- Anticipating anxiety
- Catastrophizing
- Perfectionism

AUTONOMIC NERVOUS SYSTEM

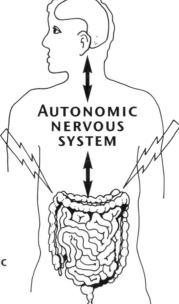

BIO-
Disruption of Colonic Smooth Muscle
- Hyperalgesia

© Copyright 2001 Paul Donovan, Ph.D.

IBS symptoms are partially due to increased sensitivity to pain in the gastrointestinal tract. It is believed that this increased sensitivity is due to changes in the rate of bowel contractions, producing experiences of pressure which are then registered as pain by the brain-gut nerve pathways. Over time, a vicious cycle develops in which the brain-gut becomes programmed to increasing sensitivity. This is called hyperalgesia—the abnormal perception of normal function, rather than the normal perception of abnormal function.

cupied with your "inside world" of body symptoms rather than the "outside world" of tension, guilt, or anger. Autonomic functioning becomes "stuck on high," leading to muscle tension, headaches, sleeping problems, lower-back pain, as well as IBS.

Because the attention is now focused inward, normal intestinal pressures and noises are perceived with anxiety, which increases the sensitivity of pain receptors. This pain-magnification process is known as

FIVE FEATURES ASSOCIATED WITH SELF-DEFEATING PATTERNS OF THINKING AND BEHAVING

Intrusive

These thoughts are obsessive; you have little control (or choice) over them. Like unwanted guests at a party, these thoughts intrude into consciousness without an invitation, and won't leave when asked.

Anticipatory

You have difficulty enjoying the pleasures of the present moment, and spend an enormous amount of time looking into the future, anticipating what may happen, then worrying about it. This is also called "thought rumination."

Catastrophic

You imagine a series of worst case scenarios: "What will happen if (this thing) occurs? I need to prepare myself for the worst now, otherwise I won't be able to cope." Your inner life is saturated with the dire images of potential threats, demands, and unpredictable events.

Perfectionist

The fear of catastrophe drives the need for perfection. Your self-imposed expectations require you to regard all tasks as equally urgent and in need of immediate attention so that they are performed totally and perfectly. The drive for perfection makes a tyranny out of time management, which further increases anxiety. At the same time, you overestimate the demands and underestimate your abilities: "It's all too much. I'll never be able to do my job. I'll never catch up. I'm useless."

Hidden

These self-defeating thought patterns become so automatic and rigid that they shape the way you respond to situations. At the same time, you remain largely unaware of the irrational distortions in your thinking processes. In fact, self-defeating thought patterns have power over behavior because they are mostly unconscious and go unrecognized.

© Copyright 2001 Paul Donovan, Ph.D.

hyperalgesia, and frequently occurs with chronic pain disorders. The person becomes very sensitive to changes in bodily sensations, and any such changes are quickly associated with a fear reaction, called somatophobia. (This is why some people are extra sensitive to medications that change bodily sensations received by the somatosensory cortex of the brain—the so-called pain threshold.) At the same time, the onset of severe IBS symptoms may help to avoid unpleasant circumstances since other people may be reluctant to upset you. If your unconscious "sick role" is successful in avoiding situations, then your IBS symptoms receive positive reinforcement. But the symptoms then become worse, establishing a vicious cycle of pain and reinforcement.

Conflict can only be avoided temporarily, however. Because the symptoms serve to repress the conflict, the failure to resolve the conflict maintains the symptoms. Most of the time, the escalating pattern of inward retreat and "sick role" reinforcement happens automatically. In fact, the pattern becomes more powerful because you are not consciously aware of what is happening.

IBS Symptoms Have Rewards

In cognitive behavioral therapy, the IBS sufferer is encouraged to consider how his or her particular self-defeating behavior is maintained and reinforced by "rewards." After all, if such patterns were totally self-defeating, they would never have become established in the first place. Such behavior enables a person to stay in control of the demands, fears, and losses of life.

For example, hypervigilance and anticipatory anxiety have "survival" value—they can contribute to high levels of performance at university, the workplace, or at home. The IBS symptoms that result from these behaviors—abdominal pain, diarrhea, constipation, etc.—may also serve a purpose: to provide unconscious "alibis" for not working, not having sex with a spouse, or not going outside the home to socialize.

From my experience in treating IBS sufferers, I find that patients often actively resist changing their automatic patterns of thinking and behaving. On the one hand, they insist on wanting to get rid of the "out-of-control" symptoms; but on the other hand, if the symptoms dissipate, they must confront what they cover up. This is their dilemma: "If I want my symptoms to reduce, then I must have the motivation to change how I think and act in my daily life, despite the advantages offered by my present coping style."

Dilemmas are really lose-lose situations in which a person is faced with conflicting choices, and each choice means a loss or punishment, usually followed by guilt or shame. It is not surprising that a person is often "paralyzed" by dilemmas in personal relationships. When this happens, the distress of the conflict may be denied by shifting it from the interpersonal arena to the body.

Most IBS sufferers struggle to avoid the choice presented by this dilemma; they also struggle to avoid recognition that there is a choice. Biomedical and dietary treatment approaches can be used as a means of avoiding the dilemma. It's much easier to change external diet than it is to change internal coping styles. An exclusive emphasis on diet keeps the problem "out there." The symptoms remain chronic despite an improved diet because the thinking and behavior patterns that created them are perpetuated. Consider the case of Joan, a 51-year-old hair stylist who had married Larry, 44, three years ago.

This was Joan's second marriage, and she had two adult children from the previous marriage. It was Larry's first marriage. While Joan found Larry to be a caring, responsive companion, she was aware from the beginning of their relationship that Larry seemed to be hostile towards her two children. Whenever the children (and young grandchildren) came to visit their mother, Larry would stay by his wife's side and adopt a sullen, withdrawn mood. He would only join the conversation to be critical of the children. Soon after they were married, a heated argument occurred between Larry and Joan's daughter that ended when the daughter cut short her overnight stay and left. The daughter then called her mother to tell her that though she loved her very much, it was impossible to visit her at her home. Larry wanted Joan for himself alone.

Joan tried but found that she couldn't confront Larry with his unreasonable behavior. She loved seeing her children, and became resentful of his jealous behavior. Joan had a long history of avoiding conflict, however, and was terrified of losing Larry if she raised the matter with him. She had been single for many years and, apart from Larry's problem with the children, she was very happy in her new relationship. This was Joan's dilemma. At the same time, she realized that her failure to declare her true feelings was driving a wedge between Larry and herself. Joan knew that Larry loved her, and reasoned therefore that she should trust that love by expressing her feelings. Rather than Larry, was it she who was betraying the relationship by keeping silent? The more Joan thought about it, the more confused she became. One minute she felt angry at Larry; in the next moment, she was overcome by guilt.

All this time, Joan's IBS symptoms were becoming worse. She had always had a "spastic colon," but the cramping, gas, and bloating were so uncomfortable now that she imagined it could only be colorectal cancer. She consulted doctor after doctor, but despite many invasive procedures and negative results, Joan remained convinced that she was going to die. She became resentful of doctors' advice, and spent her leisure time focusing on her symptoms, reading self-help books, and trying treatment after treatment. Joan's fear of a painful death now enabled her to avoid her unpleasant feelings of anger and guilt.

Meanwhile, Larry became very supportive, and was willing to share her restricted diet, and agoraphobic lifestyle. He even offered to stay with his brother on one or two occasions if her children wanted to visit. But this really didn't resolve Joan's dilemma: "How can I choose between my husband and my children?"

In Joan's case, the cognitive component of therapy was directed towards exposing this fundamental dilemma, and the fear of conflict that lay behind it.

Anxiety and IBS

Anxiety and worry are normal human emotions. They have survival value by activating the whole body and mind of the individual to meet the demands of everyday life. Anxiety enables us to prepare for examinations, to deliver a stimulating speech, to achieve project deadlines, to perform well in athletics, or many other ways of achieving our full potential.

Chronic anxiety, however, can disrupt performance as well as trigger a broad range of psychophysiological complaints, including IBS. When anxiety and vigilance develop into an habitual, apprehensive response which becomes difficult to turn off, then an individual may be suffering from an anxiety disorder. Apart from depression, there are four types of anxiety disorders commonly found among IBS sufferers. An individual may have one or more of them. They are:

Panic disorder—characterized by sudden attacks of intense fear, with physical symptoms that may include chest pain, palpitations, or chills. Panic attacks are often associated with specific situations, such as airports or shopping centers.

Phobias—including social phobia, the fear of speaking in public; agoraphobia; and food phobia, which is the progressive and excessive narrowing of diet to avoid fearful symptoms, resulting in significant weight loss.

Obsessive-compulsive disorder—characterized by persistent, inflexible thoughts regarding the completion of tasks and priorities; preoccupation with details and strict standards; and excessive devotion to work.

Generalized anxiety disorder (GAD)—unrealistic nervousness about finances, health, career prospects, or children, often resulting in stomach trouble, insomnia, and other ills, and lasting more than six months. GAD and autonomic hyperactivity are different names for the same disorder depending upon whether the diagnosis is made by a psychologist or a physician. Among the anxiety disorders, GAD is the predominant psychological diagnosis for IBS patients, and requires that at least six of the following symptoms are present. (Note that the presence of these symptoms does not always indicate GAD, and a person should consult with his or her physician to exclude hyperthyroidism and excessive consumption of coffee.)

MOTOR TENSION

- trembling, twitching, or feeling shaky
- muscle tension, aches, or soreness
- restlessness
- easily fatigued

AUTONOMIC HYPERACTIVITY

- shortness of breath or smothering sensations
- palpitations or accelerated heart rate
- sweating, or cold clammy hands
- dry mouth
- dizzy or light-headed
- nausea, diarrhea, or other abdominal distress

- flushes (hot flashes) or chills
- frequent urination
- trouble swallowing or "lump in throat"
  ### VIGILANCE AND SCANNING
- feeling keyed up or on edge
- easily startled
- difficulty concentrating or "mind going blank"
- trouble falling or staying asleep
- irritability

The IBS sufferer with GAD may have behavioral problems with children, relationship difficulties, or grief about a death in the family in the months or years preceding acute symptoms. A range of medications is available to treat all forms of anxiety, but to uncover the underlying causes and alleviate IBS symptoms, the four-step method of cognitive behavioral therapy is the treatment of choice. Let's look at how anxiety and IBS symptoms were treated in a person with a perfectionist cognitive style.

The Perfectionist IBS Profile

Bob was a 35-year-old highly paid executive in a Fortune 500 telecommunications company. He suffered from alternating diarrhea and constipation, cramping and bloating, and was very conscious of the passing of gas, which seemed to be getting worse every week. He also had chronic headaches, nausea, sinus problems, general fatigue, and muscle aches and pains all over his body.

When his internist suggested that Bob's major problem may be his hectic lifestyle, Bob came to see me. His worst symptoms occurred in the morning before work, at night or over the weekend. If it was stress, Bob reasoned to himself, then his symptoms would surely occur during the day when his load was heaviest. If it was only stress, why did the doctors keep on ordering more medical tests? Bob tended to avoid leisure activities, because that's when his symptoms were worse, but this only drove him further into his hectic work schedule.

Bob had transferred from Atlanta five years ago to take up a new position in Denver. He was on a corporate "fast-track" and the new position offered a great leap forward in his career, with a greater load of accountability. Though he would never acknowledge it, Bob was like his father, who had retired as the CEO of a telecommunications company. Although Bob had never felt close to his father, who was very strict, their relationship was important to him. His father died of colorectal cancer soon after Bob's transfer to Denver.

While Bob had always taken his good health for granted, he now started to worry about it. His three children were in middle school, and he worried about what would happen to them if he got a serious illness. His wife Joan had allowed her own career to lapse so that she could care for the children.

Bob commenced regular health checks with his doctor, stopped smoking, watched his diet, and bought an exercise machine for his basement. His new health-consciousness made a lot of sense to Bob: he knew that he had a stressful job, with long hours, and deadlines that required the cooperation of his staff. He found that he spent much of his time coaching them on simple tasks, and he became frustrated with their lack of initiative. He was a perfectionist with high standards and he expected the same of other people.

Bob remembered that his father had also complained of problems with diarrhea, constipation, and fatigue before his diagnosis of colorectal cancer. Only a year previously, a close friend and colleague in the company had died of a heart attack at work, and Bob's mother and older brother also had heart problems. Bob was always a light sleeper, but there were many nights now when he would wake up in the middle of the night and worry about things.

Not long after his transfer, Bob began to have loose bowel movements soon after he rose to go to work. He would go to the toilet several times after breakfast, and was afraid that he would soil himself at the office. Sometimes on the way to work, he experienced the urgency for a bowel movement and he would pull off the freeway to find a store with conveniences. Bob's primary-care physician checked Bob's heart, took

THE DIFFERENCE BETWEEN PERFECTIONISTS AND HIGH ACHIEVERS

Perfectionists are driven by the fear of failure:	High achievers are challenged by the opportunity to succeed:
• Set high standards	• Set high standards
• Failure means alienation and self-blame, often with depression	• Failure means disappointment
• Little satisfaction in task achievement	• High satisfaction in task achievement
• Rigid adherence regardless of the situation	• Flexible and accepting of less precision, given the situation
• Completion of tasks postponed due to repetitive checking and procrastination to avoid less than perfect performance	• Completes tasks
• Constant doubt about ability to perform	• Confident about ability to perform
• Often highly intelligent	• Often moderately intelligent
• Tries to overcome all negative moods: "If I experience a negative mood, that means there's something wrong with me."	• Comfortable with a range of moods
• Performance must be perfect or it's worthless: "A small mistake is total failure."	• Performance is balanced according to available time and resources
• A compliment is a trigger for self-criticism: "I can always do better."	• Enjoys compliments and praise: "I'm glad you like my work. I enjoyed the challenge—it stretched me."

blood samples and stool specimens, as well as X rays, but all the medical tests were negative. The doctor prescribed acid-blocker medication, but this only made Bob more nauseated.

Then he was sent to an internist, who performed a colonoscopy without detecting any abnormality. Antispasmodics were prescribed, but Bob stopped them after a few weeks. A high fiber diet seemed to provide some help. It was only when Bob went on vacation that his symptoms improved after the first few days, but they quickly returned as soon as the vacation was over. The doctors couldn't find anything wrong, and this lack of explanation only made the situation worse. Bob was becoming anxious about his body and he regarded any physical sensation as a symptom.

Then a new symptom appeared: Bob was giving a presentation to a room full of important clients, when suddenly sounds in the room became muffled. His mind went totally blank and he could feel his heart beating faster, with all these strangers' eyes looking at him. He remembered feeling light-headed, very cold and sweaty, and thought that he was having a heart attack. He felt he had to get out of the room immediately, and in the middle of his presentation, he had to hand it over to a surprised junior staff member.

In the weeks that followed, his chest pains got worse and one night his wife drove him to the hospital emergency room. But all the tests were negative. Bob became depressed and withdrawn, even within the family he loved, and his interest in sex disappeared entirely. Bob starting having arguments with his oldest son who, according to Bob, was wasting his time with losers rather than getting on with his studies. Bob felt he was dying, despite all the doctors' tests, and every day was an ordeal to keep control of his work, his fears of disapproval, and his bowels. The more out of control he felt, the greater the pressure he applied to himself.

Despite Bob's senior position, he was driven by a fear of failure, to avoid the judgment of others. He prided himself on his industry knowledge and his "Mr. Fix-It" reputation. He was always concerned that his customers were happy and made sure that he followed every project carefully, even though he was in charge of 200 employees. If anything went wrong, it was up to him to fix it while others looked on. Everything was equally important, and had to be done immediately and perfectly.

Because he monitored everything so closely, people came to him more and more often for simple decisions. He seemed to live his whole workday in a buzz of adrenaline, with people from all directions wanting his advice, while he never got around to the long-term important (but not urgent) items on his "To-Do" list. A great amount of time was spent checking and rechecking his own reports and those of his staff. At the same time, Bob was always trying to please others and constantly worried about what others thought of him. Clearly, Bob was trapped in his own patterns.

Changing Patterns Improves Health

In therapy, Bob and I talked about how behavioral and lifestyle changes could improve his health. To be able to make these changes, I explained that he needed to become aware of his habitual and automatic thought patterns. Several sessions of cognitive therapy enabled Bob to practice the following behavioral controls, in which he:

- Practiced the golden rule for perfectionists: All work is completed at the workplace during regular work hours, or else it is not completed.
- Coached others to solve their own problems, instead of taking over their work. This allowed Bob more time during the day to complete his own tasks.
- Stopped taking on tasks that he could not accomplish during regular work hours. Instead, he delegated tasks to others.
- Performed "triage" on his tasks to stop the "tyranny of the urgent," realizing that the immediately urgent tasks are not the most important tasks for the long-term.
- Stopped repetitively reviewing tasks, which diminished his obsession about mistakes and the perception that others demanded a level of performance he could not attain.

All of these changes allowed Bob to take time for strategic thinking and planning, and perform better in his assigned role—that of a senior supervisor. Bob's family life improved. He stopped taking work home and spent more time with his children. He became aware that he was re-peating an inter-generation pattern with his oldest son that he himself had experienced with his father, who was overly strict and critical. He and his wife began family conferences with the children, and started to go out on dates as a couple. And importantly, Bob's IBS symptoms sig-nificantly decreased.

Bob's perfectionism is only one of the several self-defeating cognitive behavioral styles that I have encountered in working with IBS sufferers over many years. The self-sacrificing, masochistic but passive-aggressive style is another. What's common to all these styles is the experience of anxiety and mood disturbances, and a sense that life is a constant strug-gle to keep control in the face of overwhelming demands, expectations, and traumas.

As this chapter has pointed out, such cognitive-behavioral patterns are not only problems of the mind—they are accompanied by profound physiological changes. Instead of asking which comes first, mind or body, recent research in psychobiology tells us that this mind-body rela-tionship is a complex interaction which expresses itself in a unique way for each individual. It is the challenge of the cognitive behavioral thera-pist to help individuals become aware of their unique psychophysiolog-ical patterns. And it is the challenge of IBS sufferers to confront their own unique dilemmas and regain a sense of control in their lives. Rephrased in the words of our "pop" culture: "No deposit, no return."

CHAPTER 10

The Importance of Proper Exercise

Often my IBS patients are puzzled when I encourage them to become more physically active, suggesting that this will help improve their digestive symptoms. They ask, "How will exercise help my bowels?"

Skip is a single graduate student. He came for help with classic digestive problems. His symptoms had begun a year before, and they consisted of constipation and cramping abdominal pains, with brief periods of diarrhea. Now, Skip struck me as being an easygoing intellectual type.

During our first interview, I learned that his dietary habits were atrocious. He subsisted on coffee, doughnuts, and fast food. He was almost proud of the fact that he could visit all the area's fast-food vendors and just order "the usual." Overcoming his initial skepticism, Skip began improving his diet and admitted he felt better. He still suffered periods of cramps and constipation but was basically satisfied with his progress. It was at this point that I recommended he increase his physical activity.

Skip offered countless reasons not to increase his activity. He thought the fitness craze was "just another yuppie trend. Besides, I don't have the time. I never liked exercise. I may start when I finish my thesis." And so on.

Finally, after additional inducement, Skip began incorporating some simple exercises into his daily schedule. During a follow-up visit, he commented, "I have not been constipated in months. Every morning I

114

take a brisk walk, and this seems to facilitate a bowel movement." He was very surprised to learn exercise could stimulate bowel activity. It was obvious to me he had never walked a dog.

The Benefits of Exercise

Exercise is one of the elements of a total lifestyle program to help achieve and maintain good health. Exercise helps reduce stress by providing an outlet for aggressive impulses, because stress hormones tend to dissipate during periods of increased physical activity. It makes sense that when your "fight or flight" response is triggered, exercise is an excellent way to neutralize this reaction.

In addition to helping alleviate digestive symptoms, there are other potential benefits of regular exercise. These include lessening of fatigue by improved physical endurance; increased flexibility, mobility, and strength of the musculoskeletal system; lowered cholesterol and triglyceride levels; and improved posture, appearance, and general self-image. A regular fitness program may save you money in the long run. Exercise can reduce both the need for medication and visits to the doctor about your digestive symptoms, your high blood pressure, or your diabetes. Those who are physically fit find they are less susceptible to injury and disabilities, such as lower back pain, tendonitis, and sprains. Regular exercise will have a positive impact on all aspects of your life.

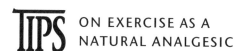

TIPS ON EXERCISE AS A NATURAL ANALGESIC

Endorphins, naturally occurring morphine-like analgesics, are released after prolonged and continuous exercise. This phenomenon seems to account for the so-called runner's high. It also explains why some people actually become addicted to exercise, braving all types of undesirable weather to get their fixes.

What to Know Before You Begin

This chapter provides information about exercise in general and some suggestions for finding a program that is right for you. For most people, there is little risk if you begin with less vigorous exercises, gradually increasing your activity level. However, if you are over 30, it is best to have your physician obtain a history and perform a physical exam, especially if you have a pre-existing medical condition. An exercise stress test (an electrocardiogram taken during exercise) may be a good idea, too, depending upon your age, heart disease risk factors, previous level of activity, and other criteria. The exercise stress test is also a helpful tool for your physician or an exercise specialist to use when assessing your most appropriate exercise intensity, based on your maximum attainable heart rate.

In most instances, your body will alert you to potential problems resulting from overdoing it. The old "no pain, no gain" or "do it until it hurts" clichés are dangerous concepts to apply to exercise. If you begin to experience dizziness, palpitations, breathing difficulties, chest pains, or muscle or joint pains, slow down or stop altogether. Chest pains and breathing difficulties are especially worrisome symptoms, as they may be early signs of cardiovascular disease, warranting medical evaluation. Always consult your doctor for advice specific to your particular situation.

You'll find your first challenge is to change your attitude towards a lifestyle that includes regular exercise. We live in a society that emphasizes economy of motion. We use elevators, escalators, shuttle buses, power steering, power brakes, and many other labor-saving devices. So begin your attitude adjustment by increasing your caloric expenditure during your normal daily activities. For example, take the stairs rather than the elevator; park farther away and walk instead of looking for the closest parking spot. With these "mini-exercises" you will burn extra calories throughout the day.

Choosing the Type of Exercise to Do

What type of exercise is best for you? There are three basic forms of exercise that contribute to maintaining health. The first type includes those that improve tone and strengthen the musculoskeletal system. These are stretching exercises, calisthenics, yoga, tai chi, and weight training. I personally like to perform some simple stretching exercises for about 20 minutes each morning. "Wake up call" for me is usually the same time each day, so, once established, this routine is easy to keep. I find it a great way to help start the day, and most people can find some time in the morning to exercise, even if it means getting up a little earlier. In addition, you may not need as much sleep as before, as you begin to experience the increased energy from your new exercise program.

Aerobic exercise is the second type of exercise to include in your program. It consists of any prolonged, rhythmical activity that uses major muscle groups. This is the type of exercise you most often hear about. Aerobic exercises require oxygen and lead to improved cardiovascular fitness. It is a way to indirectly exercise the heart and lungs. Any activity that sufficiently increases heart and respiratory rates may be considered a form of aerobic exercise. Their key requirement is movement from one point to another, and these movements include jogging, brisk walking, swimming, climbing stairs, and bicycling. Of all aerobic activities, swimming is probably the most nearly ideal: it improves aerobic fitness, while at the same time increasing overall muscle tone, without placing excessive stress on your joints. Exercises that use several muscle groups, such as swimming and using rowing machines, cross-country skiing machines, and stationary bicycles with arm levers, will burn more calories per unit of time than other types of exercise, while also improving the tone and flexibility of both the upper and lower body. You can see how certain types of exercise promote increased cardiovascular as well as increased musculoskeletal fitness.

Walking is an excellent, often underappreciated means of exercise. You may be surprised to learn that you burn just as many calories (approximately 100) by walking a mile as you do jogging a mile. Walking is a less vigorous form of aerobic exercise and is particularly well suited for elderly people, or those just beginning an exercise program. A good pair of walking or jogging shoes is all the equipment required. Weight-bearing exercises such as walking and jogging (in contrast to swimming) have the added benefit of strengthening bones, which helps to prevent osteoporosis.

My own bias is that jogging should be reserved for those who pursue it regularly. Occasional vigorous running may lead to musculoskeletal aches and pains (such as knee pain, shin splints, and bursitis). There is evidence that if you jog regularly, your musculoskeletal system adapts, lessening the possibility of adverse consequences. Again, the key is to start slowly and build up to longer distances and faster times.

It is a good idea to try combining different types of aerobic exercises, something frequently referred to as cross-training. For example, you may choose to walk or swim when weather permits, and work out on a stationary exercise bike indoors when the weather is bad. You may be interested in joining one of the wide variety of exercise classes such as aerobic dance or jazzercise. This is a good way to obtain support and encouragement and, at the same time, meet new people.

The third type of exercise includes recreational or skill activities, such as tennis, golf, racquetball, or hiking. Your calisthenic and aerobic activities should provide your basic staple of physical activity, allowing you to enjoy recreational activities even more. Additionally, these recreational activities provide another avenue for social engagement while further enhancing physical, mental, and social well-being.

Duration, Frequency, and Intensity of Exercise

As well as the best types of exercise, there are also the questions of duration (how long), frequency (how often), and intensity (how hard). Most fitness professionals recommend aerobic exercise for a minimum of 20 to 30 minutes, three or four times a week, to achieve and maintain proper cardiovascular fitness. Begin slowly with 5 to 10 minutes of exercise. Progress gradually as you increase, at a rate of one to two minutes every four or five workout sessions, or as you find you can tolerate the increase. Brief periods of warm-up and cool-down right before and after each session are advisable. During these periods, you should perform the activity at a very low level of intensity, or walk briskly in place for a few minutes.

The recommendations regarding type, duration, and frequency of exercise are relatively straightforward. But how hard should you exercise? Traditionally, the exercise intensity has been based on target heart rate zones, and the target pulse is used to determine the average rate at which you should perform the desired exercise. The target heart rate zone is usually between 60 and 85 percent of the maximum predicted heart rate (MPHR).

Without a pulse meter, it may be cumbersome to check your pulse during exercise. For this reason, the Rate of Perceived Exertion (RPE) Scale has been developed. This is a subjective estimate of exercise intensity and can be closely correlated to target pulse rates. We routinely introduce this concept to people undergoing exercise stress testing to prescribe an appropriate intensity of exercise.

When you achieve your predetermined pulse rate, decide where you are on the scale. There is no correct answer, since each person will have a slightly different perception of how hard he or she is working. The response is usually around the middle of the scale. If you rate yourself as in the range of four to six, this corresponds quite well to an appropriate exercise intensity, regardless of your age or previous activity level. The idea is to get a feeling for the appropriate intensity of exercise. Many find this concept useful when later exercising on their own, thus avoiding the need to monitor pulse rate.

As your cardiovascular fitness level improves, you will find you are able to exercise more vigorously while still maintaining your previous target pulse rate and level of perceived exertion. Your heart has become more efficient. In many (or most) IBS cases, your digestive tract will begin to function more effectively.

Your degree of breathlessness is another gauge of exercise intensity. If you are unable to speak without gasping for breath between each word, you are working too hard. In contrast, if you are able to sing the national anthem with perfect breath phrasing, you are proceeding too slowly. You should be able to carry on a conversation that requires you to take a breath every four to five words.

TIPS ON HOW TO CALCULATE YOUR APPROXIMATE MPHR

Subtract your age from 220. As an example, the MPHR of a 30-year-old person is 220 − 30 = 190. For those in poor shape, or those who primarily want to lose weight, a target pulse rate of 60 to 70 percent of your MPHR would be appropriate. In this case, the target heart rate for our hypothetical 30-year-old would be 114 to 133. If you are in poor physical condition, it may take a while for you to maintain your target pulse for the desired 20 to 30 minutes. Remember, you did not reach your present state of unfitness overnight, so be patient. Keep trying, and eventually you will reach your fitness goal.

RATE OF PERCEIVED EXERTION (RPE) SCALE

0: None
1: Very, very light
2: Very light
3: Moderate
4: Somewhat hard
5: Hard
6: Harder
7: Very hard
8: Very, very hard
9: Extremely hard
10: Maximum

The idea of exercise intensity is often difficult to grasp. Whether you use target pulse rate, level of perceived exertion, or degree of breathlessness, ask yourself at the midpoint of your routine, "Can I continue my present level of exertion for at least 15 to 20 more minutes?" If the answer is no, then you are probably working too hard.

I have counseled many patients who overdo it when beginning an exercise program. The resulting aches and pains only discourage further exercise. If you incorporate regular exercise into your lifestyle, you will, with time, begin to realize all potential benefits. You will be in better physical condition to participate in other recreational activities. In addition, you will be able to live a more active and more healthful life as you grow into your "golden years." I encourage each of you to seek guidance from your physician, an experienced trainer, or various books before launching wholeheartedly into a new lifestyle that includes regular exercise.

CHAPTER 11

Supporting Your Significant Other with IBS

IBS CAN AFFECT all aspects of an individual's life. As is true for many chronic and recurring medical conditions, the consequences of IBS will naturally affect all those close to an IBS sufferer. Living in harmony takes understanding.

If you have IBS, you may have a "significant other" who can benefit from reading this chapter to understand how you suffer. If you are the significant other without IBS, this chapter will explain this disorder, how it can affect your relationship, what you can expect from treatment, and what your partner may be doing to cope with the problem. With better understanding, you may be able to develop the support necessary to see your significant other through an IBS attack and adjust your lifestyle to ease symptoms.

For example, you're traveling down the freeway to visit Aunt Sarah. Your significant other politely requests that you take the next exit and find a rest room, and you do not. The next request is not quite so polite, because IBS turns normally compelling desires into urgent ones. As one patient remarked to me, "I don't need the next bathroom—I need the last one!"

IBS is one of those disorders employees are unlikely to report, simply because employees are embarrassed to blame absenteeism or tardiness on their bowels. One case illustrates this point. A supervisor directed a sympathetic inquiry to my office, wanting to know why one of her subordinates was getting so many "viruses." Could that worker have AIDS? I politely pointed out that I was not at liberty to discuss a patient's medical problem, but I did mention to my patient that I had received a call from her supervisor.

I suggested she level with her boss and tell her that she suffers from the most common gastrointestinal affliction, one that has been estimated to affect up to 20 percent of the population. As it turned out, the supervisor admitted that she, too, suffered similar symptoms from time to time.

Ground Rules for a Harmonious Relationship

First, it is important to discuss and negotiate mutual expectations with all the parties concerned. These expectations can be about such issues as domestic chores, sexual relations, or even such simple matters as how often you will make rest room stops while on a trip. Working out these aspects of a relationship in advance, with participation from all concerned family members, is an important step in building any relationship, even without the added impact of IBS. Such a cooperative effort becomes even more important when one family member suffers from a chronic disorder like IBS. Once you have negotiated expectations in your relationship, make an effort to adhere to them, regardless of the increase or decrease in symptoms on a given day.

Next, be aware that support is a feeling and not necessarily a set of activities. As the significant other of an IBS sufferer, you may need to set limits on the kinds of actions that are required and requested in your relationship. Sometimes an IBS partner will not be aware of being emotionally supported and will seek some action or another from you to affirm your support. In this event, tell the IBS sufferer about your supportive feelings.

Finally, monitor your own level of comfort with the disorder and your level of sympathy with the IBS sufferer. If you find yourself feeling angry or unconcerned about your significant other's disorder, or should you feel entrapped by the illness, you may seek professional help from a therapist experienced in working with family issues and chronic illnesses.

Ideally, you will feel sympathy with what IBS demands of the sufferer. At the same time, you should feel comfortable in expressing your own needs, and content to not constantly demonstrate your care through overt action. Negotiate expectations with your significant other assertively and flexibly, and then follow through consistently.

What is IBS?

TIPS **FOR COPING TOGETHER WITH IBS**

- Negotiate mutual expectations.
- Express your support in words and actions.
- Avoid making IBS the focus of your lives.
- Give love and attention when he or she is feeling well.
- Monitor your own level of comfort with the disorder.
- Seek support from others or a therapist when you feel overwhelmed.

Along with establishing harmony in your relationship, you need to know more about IBS, and how your significant other can attempt to cope with it.

IBS (irritable bowel syndrome), or spastic colon, is the most common gastrointestinal affliction in North America today, so your significant other is certainly not alone. The hallmark of IBS is abdominal pain associated with an altered pattern of bowel movements. Think back to a time when you have suffered the symptoms of a gastrointestinal virus (one the medical profession refers to less than technically as the "green apple quick-step," also known as the "trots," or the "runs"). You had cramps with their resultant pain, and the embarrassment from diarrhea was also quite unpleasant. This may be true for your significant other as well.

Others may experience the abdominal pain accompanied by constipation, and still others may have bowel movements that alternate between diarrhea and constipation, and that are never "regular" or "normal." These are the symptoms that IBS sufferers experience—either constantly or sporadically.

What causes these symptoms? There are a number of triggers that provoke these unpleasant, often embarrassing symptoms. Two of the most frequent triggers are diet and emotionally stressful situations. It is most helpful to consider them both when helping to ease your significant other through an IBS attack.

People with IBS are often sensitive to certain foods. For example, it would be unwise for you to insist that your significant other sample the chocolate mousse your boss's wife prepared if she says she would rather not. She knows from past experience there will be a price to pay. Simply let her explain, "I'm sorry, but I react to chocolate," and let it go at that. Put this way, I doubt that any host would press the matter. After all, no one wants a guest to suffer a bad reaction in his or her house.

What You Can Do to Help

Your understanding and sensitivity to what your significant other is going through can help defuse a potentially emotionally stressful situation. Often the primary consideration on the mind of IBS sufferers, whether at a formal dinner, a party, or a backyard barbecue, is "Where is the bathroom?" because they never know when the need will be urgent.

It is best to be sympathetic without making IBS the focus of your lives. Doing so, although well intentioned, will only serve to focus all thought on the problem. Most will agree that if you suffer from a toothache but can find something else to occupy your mind, the pain seems less.

I experienced this firsthand when my wife and I went through a Lamaze birth preparation class. The instructor had me apply a firm, steady pressure to my wife's upper thigh to the point that she indicated it was painful and asked me to stop. We then repeated this while she was practicing the highly focused breathing techniques she had learned in the class. It was obvious to both of us that her tolerance to pain increased as long as her mind was focused on the breathing rather than on the painful pressure I was applying. (In fact, if you have been trained as a Lamaze "coach," you may be able to help talk your significant other through a series of intense cramps.)

Under most circumstances, however, it would be preferable for the sufferer to discuss her symptoms with her doctor, or to try to work things out on her own. Doing so helps her gain a sense of control over the problem. And after all, you may not always be there to offer support.

It has been suggested that recurrent abdominal pain in some chil-

dren may be the result of a learned or conditioned response to stressful situations. The special attention and
treats they receive "to make them feel better" may actually serve to perpetuate the problem. It is felt that these
very same children could grow up to develop IBS as
adults. This is not to say that their pain is not real or that
they are attempting to get attention. However, their
symptoms may be magnified when they are allowed to
become a recurring central issue. The evidence does
suggest that your significant other should receive your
love and attention not only when she is not feeling well

TIPS ON PROVIDING SUPPORT

The most helpful and appreciated
approach to your significant other
with IBS lies somewhere between
the extremes of not caring and being
overly concerned. The best tactic
is one of informed, concerned
understanding.

but also, and most importantly, on those occasions when all seems to be
going right. Relish and nurture your relationship on the good days.

As a physician, I encounter many types of spousal relationships,
from the one who "couldn't care less" to the one who is constantly concerned, almost to a fault. The first type considers another's problem to be
just that: his or her problem, and perhaps a means to get attention from
time to time. They are clearly not concerned.

The other extreme is the one from whom I often receive calls: "Why
can't something be done? Surely there are more tests. Surely there is
some medication to relieve the suffering!" In response I explain that
there are certain limitations in the practice of medicine, even today.
There is no "quick fix" or cure, and further expensive, often uncomfortable tests will serve no useful purpose. I imagine that this same person
asks his or her significant other every day: "How are you feeling today? Is
your stomach bothering you?"

From time to time, I have advised some of my patients to seek marriage or family counseling. I sense faulty lines of communication, that
IBS or other illness is only one aspect of disturbed family relationships. I
sense sometimes the existence of hidden anger or resentment, as in the
remark, "We can't even plan a trip because of her bowels..." The response to my suggestion to seek counseling is often surprise or denial:
"There is absolutely nothing wrong with our marriage. If we could just
get a handle on this spastic colon..."

The fact is, counseling would probably enhance most relationships. I know of too few perfect marriages, and crisis intervention seems to be a North American way of life. My advice: Do not wait until the relationship is on the rocks and you are ready to see an attorney to seek professional guidance. In fact, I would like to see family counseling referred to as "family workshops" or "family seminars" to help overcome the stigma attached to it. "Jane and I are attending family workshops" sounds so much more positive than "Jane and I are in counseling."

To emphasize it once more, IBS affects many aspects of marital life, not the least of which is enjoyment of sex. Studies have shown that for many women with IBS, uncomfortable intercourse is a frequent complaint. Patients have related to me: "Who wants to have sex when you're feeling gassy and bloated?" "For years, my husband thought I was having headaches...." And we have yet to learn the impact of the emotional stress such situations foster. If this seems to be a problem area, a professional sex therapist may be able to offer some helpful suggestions.

What Changes Can Be Expected from Treatment

Since IBS is considered to be a functional disorder, that is, one without a single specific cause, we must treat the symptoms. I have seen relief in those who make significant changes in diet, who exercise, and who practice stress avoidance and stress management techniques.

You may see your significant other keeping a diet diary to record foods eaten, with reactions to certain foods or food combinations. You may notice changes in social habits, such as avoiding coffee, tea, alcohol, or cigarettes. Just because your significant other suddenly gives up the 5:00 p.m. cocktail with you does not necessarily indicate a flaw in your relationship. It could very well be an attempt to discover which factors will exacerbate the symptoms. And some changes in the timing of meals and where they are eaten may also occur.

Be ready to see more fiber appear in the daily diet, along with some changes in the weekly menu, as your significant other works to produce relief from her IBS symptoms.

Your significant other may begin a program of daily exercises, too.

These may be serving a twofold purpose: helping to improve the body's overall condition and assisting in stress relief. If you have been accustomed to "couch potatoing" after a heavy meal in the evening, you may also be called on to make some social adjustments.

What You Can Hope For

Although there is no "cure" for IBS, you can still hope for control. Diet, exercise, stress reduction, and moderation in daily living all play a significant role in this. I have found that many of my patients respond favorably to a combination of treatments. And they have begun to rediscover for themselves the normal daily and social activities that may have been difficult or impossible before. What you can hope for, then, is a return to some sort of "normalcy," where the activities and events you once shared can be yours again, without the constant stigma of "Where's the bathroom?"

In conclusion, I recommend that you be sympathetic and responsive to your significant other's needs during an attack. However, in your daily relationship, do not make spontaneous sympathetic inquiries, or dwell on the subject. When he does feel the need to let you know what he is going through from time to time, be ready to listen.

Functional GI Disorders in Children and Adolescents

by Vanessa Z. Ameen, M.D.

W HEN SUSANNE was a child, she had strong stomach pains before a test at school. Her family doctor found nothing wrong, medically speaking. When her pains were intense, she cried and pleaded with her parents to let her stay home from school, but they insisted that she go to overcome her fear of tests. Twenty years later, Susanne was diagnosed with IBS.

As a teenager, Philip missed weeks of school when he had stomach pains. He was embarrassed to tell his friends why he didn't go to "sleep-overs" or weekend trips. His father had occasional episodes of diarrhea and stomach pains, usually when he had to give presentations at work. He wondered if Philip also had a nervous stomach like him, or if something else might be going on.

Until recently, we thought that children who complained of recurring abdominal pain were either pretending or had psychological problems. After the family doctor said there was nothing wrong medically, adults could only imagine that a stomachache was an avoidance behavior. Today we know better. Children with recurring abdominal pain may be suffering from functional abdominal pain, functional dyspepsia, or IBS.

Remember—the symptoms of functional disorders cannot be explained by structural, organic, or metabolic causes. But symptoms can be so severe that children and adolescents stay home from school for days or weeks, missing out on educational, social, and recreational activities. When they go to school, their symptoms can interfere with concentration and full participation.

What causes functional GI disorders in childhood? Are there genetic influences? Are children more at risk of getting IBS if their parents have it? We know now that risk factors do exist for developing functional GI disorders later in childhood or adolescence. Colic during infancy, allergies, depression, anxiety, physical or mental abuse, and a family history of functional GI disorders all may play a role. Some children appear to have a genetic susceptibility and react to stress with gastrointestinal hyperactivity, which may be carried into adulthood. In addition, children learn attitudes and behaviors from parents and caretakers. In fact, children of parents with IBS see physicians for GI symptoms more often than children of parents without IBS. This suggests that heredity, learned behavior, or both are factors in functional GI disorders in children.

Diagnosing Childhood Functional GI Disorders

Some childhood functional GI disorders accompany normal development. For example, gastroesophageal reflux or "spitting up" usually resolves in the first year of life. Toddler's diarrhea is common among young children from one to five years of age. Other disorders may be triggered by maladapted responses to normal developmental stages such as toilet training. Withholding bowel movements occurs in up to 25 percent of toddlers at the start of toilet training, but can continue into adolescence. If these functional GI disorders are not resolved, they can interfere with a child's development and affect the entire family.

The recognition of childhood functional GI disorders depends on a child's ability to describe the multiple symptoms required to make the diagnosis. While adults are able to provide enough details to the doctor, children frequently cannot. Therefore, disorders such as IBS are not commonly diagnosed in very young children. But this does not mean that these GI disorders do not exist in this age group. When they are

TIPS ON STRESS MANAGEMENT FOR CHILDREN

Stress reduction techniques that are effective for adults are equally effective for children and adolescents. If your child's GI disorder is triggered by stress, get your child involved in a few of the following activities, depending on what is most age-appropriate. (See Chapter 9 for descriptions of stress-reduction techniques.)

• regular exercise and sports
• cognitive-behavioral therapy
• biofeedback and relaxation
• hypnosis
• progressive muscular relaxation
• yoga
• massage
• visualization

suspected, only the child's main complaints are used to suggest that a functional disorder may be the problem.

If you think your child or adolescent has one of the disorders discussed below, consult your child's physician to make sure there is no organic disease or structural or metabolic abnormality. The diagnosis can often be made based on a careful history and physical examination alone. Sometimes medical tests and/or a referral to a pediatric gastroenterologist may be needed to confirm the diagnosis.

Functional Abdominal Pain

In North America, from 10 to 30 percent of children and adolescents experience recurrent abdominal pain. Children with functional abdominal pain complain mostly of pain around the belly button that is either cramping or sharp and changes in intensity. The pain may be continuous or intermittent—often the latter—and does not usually awaken the child from sleep at night. There is no consistent relationship to meals, foods, bowel movements, position, activity, time of day, medications, or dietary changes. Other symptoms may include headache, nausea, dizziness, sweating, and paleness. After organic disease and metabolic structural abnormalities have been ruled out by either a careful and detailed history and physical examination and/or diagnostic tests (see the section on IBS below), the diagnosis of functional abdominal pain is made if the pain continues beyond three months.

This functional disorder is one of the most challenging for patients and physicians to deal with because, although there is no identifiable disease or structural abnormality, the pain is very real. Some scientific evidence suggests that functional abdominal pain is associated with hypersensitivity of the gut, which is thought to be due to abnormal communication (mediated by the neurotransmitter serotonin) between the enteric and central nervous systems (see Chapter 11, "Understanding the Psychophysiobiology of IBS").

Both physical and psychological stress can cause or trigger functional abdominal pain. Physical factors include constipation, lactose intolerance, spicy foods, drugs, and the bacteria *Helicobacter pylori* that can cause gastritis. Certain personality traits such as perfectionism or overachieving are sometimes present. Family conflict, problems at school or with friends or siblings, and physical or sexual abuse can also trigger abdominal pain.

Abdominal pain may serve to divert parents' attention from conflict, or it may allow a child to avoid an activity, situation, or relationship. When this occurs, it is called "somatization," which is the use of physical symptoms for conscious or unconscious gain. Sometimes parents unwittingly contribute to somatization by pursuing exhaustive medical tests that repeatedly show negative results. (The diagnosis of functional GI disorders is no longer made after all other possibilities have been ruled out.) Parents may also promote a "sick role" by allowing absence from school, excusing a child from household duties, giving excessive attention to symptoms, and ignoring inappropriate behavior.

Functional Dyspepsia

Functional dyspepsia, also known as nonulcer dyspepsia, affects about five percent of middle school and high school students. The diagnosis can be made from the history of a specific combination of symptoms, which may include pain or discomfort centered in the upper abdomen, upper abdominal fullness, early satiety (feeling full after eating only a small amount), bloating, or nausea. Unlike IBS, functional dyspepsia does not occur with irregular bowel movements, unless both disorders are present.

When functional dyspepsia is suspected, children may be given drugs to reduce acid in the stomach. If there is no improvement in symptoms, an upper endoscopy exam may be performed by a gastroenterologist to look inside at the esophagus, stomach, and beginning part of the small intestine. Endoscopy and ultrasound may be used to make sure there is no underlying disease such as inflammatory or eosinophilic bowel disease, infection with *H. pylori,* or a food allergy.

Treatment for functional dyspepsia in children is similar to treatment for adults and includes discontinuing medications and foods known to aggravate the symptoms. The common medications used include antacids, metoclopramide, and tricyclic antidepressants (TCAs).

IBS

From 5 to 15 percent of middle school and high school students have symptoms that suggest IBS. The diagnosis of IBS, which requires a combination of specific symptoms, is usually made in adults and older children because they can describe their symptoms; younger children are usually not able to do so.

By this chapter, you know the tell-tale symptoms of IBS: recurring abdominal discomfort or pain that is relieved after a bowel movement and/or occurs with a change in frequency or form of stools. Medical tests, if deemed necessary, have ruled out inflammation, structural, or metabolic abnormalities; there is no blood in the stool, fever, pain in the joints, weight loss, or unusual skin rashes. Similar to adults, children and adolescents with IBS may suffer from alternating constipation and diarrhea, with one of these two symptoms predominating.

When IBS or functional abdominal pain is suspected, diagnostic testing (if any are performed) may include a complete blood cell count, urinalysis, testing of stool for blood and infections, a lactose breath hydrogen test, an ultrasound, X rays, or an endoscopy. It is thought that children and adolescents who are eventually diagnosed with IBS may initially have suffered from abdominal pain only.

Functional Constipation

About one in six children, both boys and girls, suffer from chronic constipation. Functional constipation causes a child to strain or feel pain from the passage of stools, which are hard and pebble-like. Bowel movements may sometimes be large enough to clog the toilet, and may occur less than three times a week. Any one of these symptoms occurring for at least two weeks points to chronic constipation. When poorly managed, it can lead to severe abdominal pain, distension, and vomiting. Functional fecal retention or enuresis (bed-wetting or the involuntary passage of urine) may also result, leading to psychological problems and absence from or failure at school.

Chronic constipation can be very worrisome to parents. If you have ever taken your child to the hospital or to a specialist for fear that there is some serious underlying disorder, you are not alone. Twenty-five percent of the visits to pediatric gastroenterologists are due to concerns about functional or chronic constipation. However, only a minority of these children are constipated due to an organic (not functional) cause.

If you suspect your child is constipated, you should know what is a normal number of bowel movements for the age of your child. During the first week of life, infants have about four stools a day, although breastfed infants may not have a bowel movement for several days or longer. By two years of age, toddlers have about one to two bowel movements a day. By four years, bowel movements have decreased to about one a day, a rate which is considered normal throughout childhood and adolescence.

There are several stages during a child's normal development when constipation is likely to occur: when breastfeeding is replaced by infant formula; when baby foods and solids are added to the diet; when whole cow's milk replaces infant formula (recommended at one year of age); at toilet training; and when a child begins school and needs to ask permission to go to the rest room. Withholding stool at the start of toilet training can lead to stools that become harder the longer they are withheld, causing painful defecation that perpetuates the withholding. For all of these developmental stages, constipation can be resolved by providing appropriate foods, fluids, and behavioral techniques.

Functional Fecal Retention and Fecal Soiling

Functional fecal retention begins when a child fears that a bowel movement will be painful. (It also tends to occur at the normal developmental stages specified for functional constipation.) Consequently, bowel movements are withheld, sometimes for weeks until finally, when they are passed, they are very large. In addition, the passing of large, hard stools can tear the anus, which may cause streaks of blood on the outside of the stool or on the toilet paper. This can be painful and frightening to both children and parents. When stool is withheld for long periods, fecal soiling may occur. This is the leaking of liquid stool around the hard mass of retained stool or leaking when gas is passed. Fecal retention can last for years because children may be ashamed and hide their soiled underwear.

The best treatment is prevention of painful bowel movements. If you are concerned that your child is withholding stool, establish fixed times for using the toilet. This practice promotes regularity. You can also reward young children for cooperation and successful bowel movements. Dietary changes and medications (listed below) help to soften the stool and prevent painful passage.

When fecal soiling occurs without fecal retention, the disorder is called nonretentive soiling. In this case, children have bowel movements at inappropriate times and places, without the problems of pain or constipation. If your child has this disorder, it is best to seek help from your child's doctor and possibly a therapist. The most common cause is an emotional or deeper psychological disturbance.

Toddler's Diarrhea

Children with toddler's diarrhea are usually healthy-looking, although they pass three to four or more liquid or loose stools a day. The stools may smell foul, contain mucus and undigested vegetable matter, and are passed earlier in the day and not at night. Children may have some abdominal pain as well. Fortunately, by three years of age, toddler's diarrhea is resolved in more than 90 percent of children. There is some evidence that adults with IBS may have had toddler's diarrhea in childhood.

Diet often plays an important role in causing toddler's diarrhea, and therefore treatment includes dietary changes. Children with this disorder usually consume low fat and fiber foods and drink excessive amounts of liquids with fructose and sorbitol. In fact, toddler's diarrhea may disappear in some children by simply increasing the fat and fiber content in their diets and limiting liquids with sorbitol.

Other factors that play a role include lack of physical activity; antibiotic usage that may disrupt the beneficial bacteria in the gut; and stress. Acute gastroenteritis or other viral infections, and possibly colic and constipation, may precede toddler's diarrhea.

Gastroesophageal Reflux

This disorder is also known as regurgitation or spitting up. It is common in infants and may be due to the immature development of the esophagus and related organs. Spitting up likely occurs when the sphincter muscle of the lower esophagus suddenly relaxes. In the first three months of life when feeding difficulties are not uncommon and accompanied by crying, refusal to breastfeed, gas, or colic, spitting up may be very worrisome to parents. By six to eight months of age when the baby can sit upright, there is more muscular coordination and spitting up decreases. It also improves when solid foods are introduced to the diet.

If spitting up or vomiting occurs with other signs, reflux disease or another structural or congenital abnormality may be the cause. In these cases, the following signs are present: vomit containing blood or bile-containing fluids, which appear yellow, green, or brown; forceful or projectile vomiting; poor weight gain; gagging; and constant irritability. Damage to the inner lining of the esophagus could be present due to stomach acid in the esophagus, a foreign body, or accidental ingestion of household poisons. There are several tests your physician can undertake to determine if spitting up is more than a developmental stage.

Before any of these tests are necessary, parents can manage normal gastroesophageal reflux by following these simple techniques—after you have sought the advice of your child's physician:
- give smaller amounts of feedings more frequently;
- thicken feedings with cereal to increase the consistency;
- and set your child upright without slouching during and after feeding to make the most of gravity.

Aerophagia

Aerophagia is the swallowing of excessive volumes of air; as a functional problem it may result from children talking too much during meals. The most common symptom is abdominal distention due to excess air or gas in the bowel, which increases during the day and becomes acute by nightfall. Associated symptoms are burping, abdominal cramps, colic, and gas. The treatment of aerophagia is largely making changes to diet and behavior: no gum chewing, no carbonated beverages, and less talking while eating.

Treating the Predominant Symptoms of GI Disorders

While the specific GI disorders that affect children and adolescents differ, several share the common symptoms of abdominal pain, constipation, and diarrhea. The following are standard and generally accepted treatments of abdominal pain, constipation, and diarrhea. But remember—consult with your physician for the right treatment that suits your child's needs and circumstances. For older children and adolescents who can report the necessary details to make a diagnosis, treatment for functional GI disorders is similar to recommendations for adults.

ABDOMINAL PAIN

Children react to pain in differing ways. Many children have an intolerance for even mild discomfort and are incapacitated by it, while others cope better and prefer to engage in activities. It's important to be aware that a child with a functional GI disorder may have increased sensitivity to pain, called hyperalgesia. Frequent and repetitive painful stimuli can sensitize the gut so much that any internal sensation will send a pain signal to the brain. It is important for both you and your child to be aware of this hypersensitivity.

Functional abdominal pain is easier to manage than eradicate. Parents, caretakers, teachers, and the suffering child all need to be reassured and educated about hypersensitivity to pain. There are links between the physical and psychological stresses in your child's life that trigger or make the pain worse; these need to be acknowledged before they can be managed. With this understanding, it is easier for your child to maintain or resume normal daily activities.

If the cause of abdominal pain is due to psychological factors, the best approach is to get help to deal with the personal or family stress. Keep in mind that recurrent abdominal pain in some children may be a learned or conditioned response to stressful situations. The special attention and inappropriate rewards received for pain may make them feel better, but it may also perpetuate the problem. As soon as you know there is no underlying disease or abnormality causing the pain, it is most effective to show concern and empathy while encouraging your child to manage the pain to be able to carry on with daily activities.

If abdominal pain results from, or is made worse by food intolerances or sensitivities, then consider the dietary recommendations discussed below and in Chapter 5, "Tracking Down Problem Diet Factors." Sometimes simply eliminating problem foods such as caffeine or milk products will put an end to the pain.

There are some medications that have proven effective in treating abdominal pain in children and adolescents. TCAs in lower doses than those used for depression have analgesic effects and may be of some benefit in treating functional abdominal pain. However, the different TCAs have varying side effects that need to be taken into account when individualizing treatment.

CONSTIPATION

The treatment for constipation depends on its severity. If it is chronic and stools are impacted, treatment may take place in stages, beginning with giving medicines to clean out stools in the large intestines. If constipation is intermittent, improving the diet and bowel habits may be all

TIPS FOR HELPING CHILDREN COPE WITH ABDOMINAL PAIN AT SCHOOL

If the doctor recommends that your child return to school and cope with abdominal pain, it is important to develop a consistent home and school pain management strategy. Ask your child's teachers and school staff to be sympathetic about the pain, but not allow it to affect attendance or performance. If teachers are not able to cope with symptoms when they significantly disrupt the class, work out a temporary measure of partial school attendance or homeschooling. The key is consistency and collaboration.

that is needed. However, it is often necessary to give some form of medication to maintain bowel regularity, because until this occurs, relapses are common.

The stages for relieving chronic constipation are as follows. To relieve impacted stools in the rectum, glycerine suppositories may be given to infants and enemas given to children over one year of age. Giving medications by mouth (such as magnesium citrate, magnesium hydroxide, mineral oil, and PEG solution) may also be used to relieve impaction.

When stools are loosened and eliminated, then improving bowel habits and diet can begin. Non-stimulant laxatives such as mineral oil, lactulose (well tolerated over the long-term), and sorbitol (less expensive than lactulose) may be needed to keep the stools soft. Stimulant laxatives should be used only in an acute case and otherwise avoided. Consult your child's doctor before starting any treatment to make sure that your child receives appropriate care.

TIPS ABOUT MEDICATIONS FOR CHILDREN WITH FUNCTIONAL GI DISORDERS

There are few clinical studies of medications for children and adolescents for most diseases, including the functional GI disorders. The current research on drugs for IBS, targeting the sensory and motor malfunctions of the enteric nervous system, are for adults. Many drugs given to children are based on projections from adult studies. We need much more medical research dedicated to the needs of children.

Reviewing your child's diet is always important in treating constipation, whatever the form. Make sure your child eats four or more servings of fresh fruit, vegetables, and whole grains daily. Keeping a daily diet diary may prove to both you and your child that important foods are lacking, while others may be triggers of abdominal pain and constipation.

A diet deficient in fiber is a known contributor to constipation. Adding fiber to decrease constipation may not necessarily be difficult, with the range of whole grain breads and high fiber cereals available. To determine how many grams of fiber to add to your child's diet, simply add the number five to your child's age; the result is the grams of fiber needed daily. Increasing liquid intake is also essential; include juices higher in sorbitol and fructose such as prune, pear, and apple juice.

As mentioned earlier, establishing a regular time to use the toilet can result in regular bowel movements. This is best done by having the child sit on the toilet after meals, which is when the intestines are most active. It is best to practice this after breakfast to establish a pattern for the day.

DIARRHEA

The treatment of diarrhea, whether it is toddler's diarrhea or a symptom of IBS, is generally focused on eliminating problem foods and improving the diet. For toddlers and older children, the problem foods are fruit drinks and juices high in fructose and sorbitol (especially apple and pear juice) and candies containing sorbitol. For both age groups it is also important to increase foods with fiber and higher fat content, which is done by simply avoiding low-fat foods. While there is no evidence that adding fiber decreases diarrhea, it is important to examine the fiber content in your child's daily diet to make sure that it is adequate.

For older children and adolescents, the treatment of IBS-predominant diarrhea is similar to the treatment for adults. (See Chapter 14, "All About Medications," for more information.) For toddler's diarrhea, aspirin, psyllium, and loperamide have been found by some physicians to be useful.

A Prescription for Parents

Even though many functional GI disorders are common in childhood and accompany developmental stages, you may not be fully relieved. You still have to help manage the symptoms until they are outgrown. Unfortunately, some disorders may be perpetuated by inappropriate behaviors and require a physician and possibly a psychotherapist to resolve. You may need to give closer attention to how your family is functioning—your child may be reacting to stresses that everyone else apparently tolerates. And perhaps your family's diet needs a comprehensive overhaul.

My general recommendation is to regard these problems as an opportunity for the whole family to grow. You may have unknowingly inherited habits and beliefs about diet and pain that need to be cast off.

You may have a functional GI disorder yourself and need to deal with it. Seek professional medical help and examine your parenting skills. The changes and adaptations you make to foster your child's health may benefit you all.

This chapter is dedicated to my family who have all provided encouragement and support throughout my career, especially my father. Special thanks to Susan H. Gordon, M.S.N. and Joanne Grainger, Pharm.D. of North American Medical Affairs of GlaxoSmithKline for their review and input.

CHAPTER 13

All About Medication

A N ESTIMATED 45 to 75 percent of IBS sufferers who seek medical advice take at least one prescribed drug to find relief. Those with severe symptoms often try several combinations of drugs. So it is not surprising that physicians often ask me when I lecture, "What do you use to treat IBS?"

First and foremost, I answer, there is no substitute for a concerted effort to gain control of IBS symptoms through proper diet, stress reduction, and exercise. Secondly, when medications are used, they should be selected for the individual to treat specific symptoms. In fact, recent studies are designed to assess the effectiveness of medications in specific subgroups of IBS sufferers.

In the past, no studies demonstrated a consistent benefit for the constellation of IBS symptoms. But a comprehensive review of studies conducted over the past 30 years and published in the *Annals of Internal Medicine* (July 2000) reveals smooth-muscle relaxing drugs to be effective for abdominal pain and loperamide to be effective for diarrhea. However, the smooth-muscle relaxing drugs have not been approved for use in the United States. (See page 150 for a discussion of new medications.)

Your physician will analyze your situation to determine which, if any, medications may be most helpful. Physicians may prefer certain medications as a result of personal experience. Remember that what works for Aunt Millie may not work for you. Also remember that some people have spontaneous remission of symptoms.

What to Ask about Medication

Just as some people are anxious for medication to resolve their problems, others would rather avoid drugs under any circumstances. I respect both ends of this spectrum. With this in mind, here are my observations about IBS medication.

If your physician prescribes medication for you, make certain you get answers for the following questions:

- What is the purpose of the medication?
- How does this medication work?
- Is it habit forming?
- When should I take this medication?
- Should I take it all the time, or only when I have symptoms?
- What might happen if I suddenly stop taking the medication?
- What are the effects of long-term use?
- What are the common side effects?

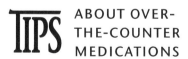 ABOUT OVER-THE-COUNTER MEDICATIONS

While many IBS sufferers do not seek help from a physician to relieve their symptoms, many do take over-the-counter drugs. If you suffer from alternating diarrhea and constipation, over-the-counter medications may contribute to these alternating symptoms.

Whenever I see a patient with any new complaint, I assess his or her use of medications (prescription and non-prescription) and supplements to see if this new complaint or constellation of symptoms started sometime after the new medication or supplement was begun. For example, high doses of vitamin C can cause diarrhea. Additionally, many medications may rarely produce untoward side effects or cause problems in an individual that aren't generally accepted or reported. Only by looking for a temporal relationship between starting something new and the development of new symptoms, can these rare so-called, idiosyncratic reactions be determined. Adverse effects produced by drug interactions may further compound the problem with the use of multiple medications (polypharmacy).

It is most important to check with your physician before taking medication prescribed by another practitioner or purchased over-the-counter to minimize harmful drug interactions. Also be aware that herbal remedies contain ingredients that, taken without a prescription, may worsen your IBS symptoms or interact with medications. Tell your physician about all the medications and herbal remedies you are taking. For example, St. John's Wort, a popular herb taken as an antidepressant, may speed up the breakdown of other medication, and has been shown to render birth control pills less effective, resulting in an unwanted pregnancy. Also, be particularly careful with alcohol. It is a common drug that may interact with a variety of medicines, usually causing excessive drowsiness, and impairing your ability to drive and safely operate hazardous equipment.

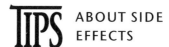

ABOUT SIDE EFFECTS

The term "common side effects" is used because it is not practical or worthwhile to inquire about all the possible side effects of a medication. Your doctor will be able to tell you which ones are fairly frequent and should be of concern to you. If, however, you begin taking a medication and all does not seem as it should be, check with your physician to see if you are experiencing an unusual side effect.

Classifications of IBS Medications

The major symptoms of IBS are abdominal pain and altered bowel habits. The goals of drug therapy are, therefore, to alleviate the pain and regularize the bowel movements. Often, if the bowel movements become more regular through dietary changes or use of fiber supplements, the pain is lessened and medications may not be needed.

When medication is needed, be aware that pharmacological treatment of any disorder must be individualized (based on a multitude of factors) by your physician. This section reviews the classes and specific agents of pharmacological medications that are most frequently used to treat IBS symptoms. It is intended to supplement, but not replace, information provided by your physician and drug manufacturer. While not an exhaustive list of all the medications available in treating IBS, it is a current update of those that have shown possible benefit in my own experience or in clinical studies. For ease of recognition, I have included both trade and generic names of agents.

Remember that any medication is capable of producing side effects. Rare individual or so-called idiosyncratic reactions may occur in susceptible people. The likelihood that anyone will experience a side effect may relate to the dose or duration of therapy. Concomitant use of other medications may increase the likelihood of experiencing an unwanted drug interaction or side effect.

A word about the use of medications during pregnancy and breast-feeding is in order. A medication intended for the mother may have adverse effects on the developing fetus or breast-feeding infant. Although the list of drugs that definitely cause fetal abnormalities is relatively short, information regarding the absolute safety of a medication is seldom available. For this reason, I would rather not recommend any medication to a pregnant or breast-feeding woman. If you are pregnant or think you may be, check with your physician about the risks and benefits of drug therapy.

Medications for Abdominal Pain and Bloating

The first and most commonly used medications prescribed for IBS treat abdominal pain and bloating. The antispasmodics relieve bloating and cramps by reducing the frequency and intensity of smooth muscle spasms in the intestines. They are best used before situations where you expect IBS symptoms to occur. Peppermint oil, by the way, is a natural antispasmodic widely used in Europe; caffeine-free peppermint tea may relieve less severe symptoms. (See Chapter 14 for information on herbal remedies.)

The antispasmodics work by inhibiting the action of nerves that regulate the intestinal smooth muscle and certain secretory glands found in the intestinal tract. Antispasmodics may be also helpful for treating symptoms associated with peptic ulcer disease, diarrhea, and diverticulosis.

Common Examples: Clidinium bromide (Quarzan), dicyclomine (Bentyl), hyoscyamine sulfate (Anaspaz, Cystospaz, Cystospaz-M, Levsin, Levsinex Timecaps), methscopalamine (Pamine).

Side Effects: The most common side effects of the antispasmodics in-

144

clude dry mouth, blurred vision, dizziness, difficulty emptying the bladder, and constipation. If you experience dry mouth, you may aggravate your symptoms by using gum or mints, or drinking excessive liquids at mealtimes in an effort to combat this side effect. Less common side effects are nervousness, anxiety, delirium, drowsiness, insomnia, rapid heartbeat, nasal congestion, rash, itching, flushing, decreased sweating (which may predispose you to heat exhaustion), and impotence.

How to Use the Medication: Antispasmodics are best taken 30 minutes before meals. Since they may cause drowsiness, caution should be used when performing tasks that require alertness. Notify your doctor if you develop any of the above-mentioned side effects, the most common of which are dry mouth, difficulty in urination, constipation, and increased sensitivity to light. Patients with glaucoma should not use antispasmodics. Eye pain may be a side effect in persons with previously undiagnosed glaucoma.

Medications for Diarrhea

Diarrhea may be defined as stools that are more frequent than usual (generally more often than three times a day) or stools that are excessively liquid. There are various causes of diarrhea, including diarrhea associated with IBS. Caution should be used when treating diarrhea associated with infections of the gastrointestinal tract, since antidiarrheal drugs may interfere with the body's attempt to get rid of the infectious agent.

Under certain circumstances, the so-called nonnarcotic opioids may be prescribed to treat troublesome diarrhea, especially "nervous diarrhea," which may occur on the first day of a new job or on a backpacking trip or another outing where frequent bowel movements may be most inconvenient. Loperamide (Imodium) has been most commonly recommended to decrease stool frequency and improve stool consistency. It slows down movement of the intestines and increases water absorption. However, it does not reduce abdominal pain and distention. Diphenoxylate, also a GI relaxant, works similarly to loperamide, but should be used with extreme caution in patients with liver disease.

Other agents used to treat diarrhea include the anti-secretory agents (Pepto-Bismol). These agents help stimulate absorption of fluids and electrolytes across the intestinal wall. The antispasmodics have been used as antidiarrheal agents, but their primary effect is to relieve cramps by reducing intestinal smooth-muscle contractions. The so-called adsorbents (Kaopectate) are thought to act by adsorbing excess water in the gastrointestinal tract. The "bile-acid sequestrants" (Colestid, Questran) relieve diarrhea that is thought to be secondary to excessive bile salts (which are produced by the liver). These agents may be particularly effective in individuals with diarrhea after having gallbladder removal (cholecystectomy).

Common Examples: Bismuth subsalicylate (Pepto-Bismol), camphorated tincture of opium (Paregoric), cholestyramine (Questran), colestipol (Colestid), diphenoxylate hydrochloride and atropine sulfate (Lomotil), kaolin and pectin (Kaopectate), loperamide hydrochloride (Imodium).

Side Effects: These vary with the different types of anti-diarrheal agents. All of these agents may cause constipation as a side effect and should not be used when diarrhea is associated with blood in the bowel movement or with fever. In addition to causing constipation, the opioids may cause nausea, vomiting, drowsiness, dizziness, nervousness, confusion, blurred vision, dry mouth, difficulty urinating, and an irregular heartbeat. Bismuth subsalicylate may cause dark stools or a dark tongue. The adsorbents are generally quite safe but may interfere with the adsorption of other medications. A two- to three-hour interval is recommended between the administration of adsorbents and the administration of other drugs.

How to Use the Medication: Your physician will need to determine the appropriate anti-diarrheal agent for you to use.

Medications for Constipation

The normal bowel movement should be neither hard nor loose and should be easily passed without straining. Constipation occurs when the stools are hard and difficult to pass. Therefore, the consistency of the

146

stool rather than the frequency of elimination determines the extent of constipation. Laxatives are frequently misused because of lack of understanding of bowel function. For example, when potent laxatives are taken, the colon may empty of all fecal material, and two or three days may be required to re-establish a sufficient quantity of fecal mass for the next bowel movement. This lag time may be perceived as constipation and more laxatives may be ingested, resulting in a vicious cycle. Further, laxatives can aggravate and contribute to the alternating symptom pattern of diarrhea and constipation.

In most instances, adequate intake of fruits, vegetables, and grains in an active individual will help maintain normal stool frequency and consistency. If these measures fail, the bulk-forming agents are the most widely used, although they take several hours to have the desired effect. These laxatives are prescribed to "normalize" the bowel movements. They work by retaining water and make a hard stool softer. While bulking agents have been commonly prescribed for treating diarrhea, current studies do not support this use.

While psyllium, methylcellulose, and bran are commonly prescribed, the agent I prefer to prescribe for constipation is calcium polycarbophil. Calcium polycarbophil tablets can be taken easily with water and do not need to be mixed with liquids; also, they do not contain sugar or artificial sugar additives, which should be avoided.

With so many products on the market for constipation, you may be wondering how your physician makes a choice. Generally speaking, I prescribe bulking agents for chronic constipation. When constipation is intermittent, I prescribe Milk of Magnesia, a so-called saline laxative. If none of these agents are effective, then I recommend osmotic laxatives, like lactulose or PEG solution. Lactulose, an osmotic laxative, may be effective for treating people with constipation-predominant IBS if other measures fail. Lactulose, which is a sugar containing lactose and galactose, works by drawing water and electrolytes into the colon, making the stool softer and stimulating contractions. Side effects include nausea, bloating, cramps, and flatulence. A new osmotic agent for treating constipation is MiraLax, a powered form of polyethylene glycol.

If none of the above agents relieve your constipation, I suggest you see a rectal specialist to make sure you do not have a mechanical problem.

Common Examples: Bulk-forming agents—calcium polycarbophil (Equalactin, Fibercon, Mitrolan), psyllium (Fiberall, Hydrocil, Konsyl, Metamucil, Perdiem), methylcellulose (Citrucel); saline laxatives—Milk of Magnesia; osmotic laxatives—lactulose (Cephulac, Chronulac, Duphulac), PEG solution, MiraLax.

Side Effects: Bulk-forming agents are usually safe when taken with adequate amounts of liquid (at least eight ounces per dose). Intestinal obstruction may occur if adequate amounts of liquid are not taken. Rare allergic reactions to psyllium products have been reported.

The initial administration of lactulose for treatment of constipation may cause excessive gas and cramps, particularly in individuals with coexisting lactose intolerance. These symptoms often improve with continued use and the establishment of regular soft bowel movements. Excessive doses may produce watery stools.

How to Use the Medication: Remember to take bulk-forming agents with adequate amounts of liquid, preferably around mealtime, so that they mix with the food. If you are overweight, take them before meals to help curb your appetite. If you are at or below your ideal body weight, take them after meals. Be patient—it may take up to 72 hours for the initial laxative effects to be noted.

Lactulose may be mixed with fruit juice or water to improve the taste. Remember, gas and cramps may occur with the initial doses. Start with a low dose and gradually increase every few days as needed.

Antidepressants

Antidepressants have shown benefit in the treatment of various chronic pain syndromes (such as low back pain, headache, fibromyalgia syndrome) and may be helpful for the chronic, recurrent abdominal pain associated with IBS. Some also possess anti-anxiety properties and may be helpful in treating IBS symptoms provoked by stress. Through mechanisms that are not clearly understood, it may turn out that antidepressants favorably affect the enteric nervous system in IBS sufferers. The tricyclics (also called TCAs) may have beneficial effects on intestinal motility and sensitivity of the gut, thereby relieving pain. Although effective for treating depression, the selective serotonin-reuptake inhibitors (SSRIs) to date have not been shown to be effective for IBS.

However they work, antidepressants are occasionally useful as part of the total treatment program for IBS. Most of them take about two to three weeks to achieve their maximum beneficial effect at any given dose. Usually therapy is begun with low doses and gradually increased every two to three weeks as needed

Common Examples: Tricyclic antidepressants—amitriptyline (Elavil), desipramine (Norpramin), doxepin (Sinequan), imipramine (Tofranil), nortriptyline (Pamelor).

Side Effects: The tricyclics are the oldest, most established class of antidepressant medication. Common side effects include dry mouth, sedation, and a hung-over feeling. These side effects usually abate with continued use. Other, less common side effects include sleep disturbance, nightmares, sweating, blurred vision, constipation, rapid heart rate, decreased blood pressure, worsening of glaucoma, and urinary retention. With long-term use, symptoms of Parkinson's disease may develop— tremor, muscle rigidity, and general slowing of muscular activity (bradykinesia). These symptoms may become apparent with abrupt withdrawal of the medication.

How to Use the Medication: Like other prescription medications, antidepressants must be taken exactly as prescribed. Allow two to three weeks before deciding whether or not they are helping. Exercise caution while driving or performing tasks that require mental alertness. Use with alcohol should be avoided, since sedation will be worsened. Dry mouth and sedation will often lessen with continued use.

Anti-anxiety Agents

Since emotional stress may precipitate IBS symptoms, the anti-anxiety, or "minor tranquilizers," are often prescribed to treat this aspect of the disorder. I advise patients to develop coping skills with assistance from a therapist, and practice self-help relaxation techniques rather than rely-ing on a particular medication to deal with life's stresses. (See Appendix 5, "Resources," for how to order the relaxation tape cassette, *Stress and IBS*.) However, these agents may be useful in treating symptoms of IBS that are clearly exacerbated by stressful situations—for example, "nerv-ous diarrhea," which some authorities believe should be considered a separate condition from IBS. But used daily on a long-term basis, these medications can cause a pattern of physical and psychological addiction to develop. As well as their being habit-forming, other potential prob-lems include over-sedation, particularly if taken with alcohol.

New Medications

In February 2000, the first of a new generation of agents was released. Alosetron (Lotronex), based on research into the connection between the central and enteric nervous systems (CNS and ENS), was found to be effective for women with diarrhea-predominant IBS. Unfortunately, the drug was voluntarily withdrawn from the market in November 2000 because of reports about its potential side effects, some of which were severe. This led to a re-evaluation of the risks versus benefits of this medication. In my opinion, when Lotronex was properly prescribed ac-cording to its indications, it was very effective for women with diarrhea-predominant IBS, whose symptoms were severe enough to adversely affect their quality of life and interfere with work and recreation.

Current medications under investigation are targeting physiological functions such as intestinal motility or visceral sensitivity. Tegaserod, a promising new medication, another agent based on CNS-ENS research, has shown benefit for the treatment of constipation-predominant IBS. Tegaserod was recently approved by the FDA and should be available sometime in 2001. For updates on new mediactions visit IBSinforma-tion.com.

Drugs targeting intestinal motility are serotonin agonists/antag-onists, CCk antagonists, selective M1 antagonists, calcium channel blockers, and alpha-2 agents. Drugs being researched to affect pain threshold in the gut are opiod-like agents and visceral pain antagonists. Research continues into antidepressants and enkephalin/endorphin analogs.

More research into medications is needed. I am encouraged that IBS has become recognized as a legitimate disorder, and that the pharmaceutical industry is actively seeking treatment options.

Digestive Aids

Food intolerances to lactose and gas-causing foods may be treated with enzyme supplements. Lactose intolerance results in gas, cramps, bloating, and diarrhea. Lactase enzyme supplements are specifically designed to break down the sugar lactose. They are used to treat milk to decrease the lactose content, or may be taken with milk or lactose-containing products. (See Appendix 3, "Lactose-Free Diet," for more information about lactose intolerance.)

BEANO is a special enzyme that breaks down the complex sugars (oligosaccharides) in many gas-causing foods, making them more digestible. BEANO works on a variety of foods (including beans, cabbage, broccoli, cauliflower, onions) by breaking down the gas-producing sugars into smaller sugar molecules that are more easily digested and ab-

IBS MEDICATIONS AND THEIR USES

	Abdominal pain	Bloating	Diarrhea	Constipation
Antispasmodics	acute, intermittent	X		
Antidepressants	chronic			
Antidiarrheals			X	
Bulking Agents				X
Laxatives				X
*tegaserod	X	X		X

*See page 150 for more information.

sorbed. If undigested these large sugar molecules enter the colon, where fermentation with bacteria produces the gas and bloating.

Common Examples: Lactrase, Lactaid, BEANO, and Dairy Ease.

Side Effects: Enzyme supplements are generally well tolerated. BEANO is made from a mold, and persons allergic to penicillin may have an allergic reaction to BEANO.

How to Use the Medication: Digestive enzymes should be taken immediately before or with meals. A few drops of BEANO should be added to the first bite or two of the offending food. It will not work at high temperatures and should be added to food that is not above 130° Fahrenheit. As a general rule, if the food is not steaming, it's all right to add BEANO.

CHAPTER 14

A Complementary Approach to IBS

by Raphael J. d'Angelo, M.D.

COMPLEMENTARY ALTERNATIVE MEDICINE (CAM) has emerged in the last decade from a trickle of idle interest to a waterfall of societal change. In 1999, a staggering $25 billion in the U.S. was spent by consumers in pursuit of CAM remedies. The National Institutes of Health has even established a department to fund and oversee the scientific investigation of CAM treatments. CAM users tend to be well educated, have an income above the national mean, and believe that the CAM philosophy of preventive care and self-healing fits into their own world view. It is no wonder then that some IBS patients have sought out CAM therapies rather than go first to a traditional doctor.

Some CAM modalities that have been used to treat IBS are acupuncture, chiropractic, traditional Chinese medicine, Ayurveda, aromatherapy, herbal therapy, homeopathy, biofeedback, and meditation. Many of these therapies manipulate the body's energy according to Eastern systems of health care. They see the human organism as an interconnected whole. Western traditional healers are taught that the body is the sum of separate, compartmentalized organs and tissues; the emphasis is to diagnose a disease and fix the part that is sick.

As a holistic family physician, I use CAM in my practice. I have studied the literature regarding nutritional, herbal, and aromatherapeutic techniques and use them when I can for the relief of IBS. Nutritional therapy uses foods, vitamins, and minerals the way traditional therapy uses drugs. Herbal therapy involves the use of various herbal preparations to achieve relief or healing. Aromatherapy (also known as aromatic medicine) is the administration of potent plant oils usually by mouth or inhalation to cause immune and chemical changes in the body.

The CAM Dietary Approach

In CAM treatment, proper diet is most important, and this subject has been thoroughly presented in earlier chapters. CAM therapies agree that food intolerance is a major factor in some IBS patients. In these individuals, dramatic improvement can be noted with an elimination diet. Cow's milk and dairy products lead the list of frequent food offenders. The presence of yeast in the intestinal tract of a food sensitive person will enhance the adverse food reactions. Also, the neuroexcitory amino acids MSG and aspartame (Nutrasweet) may exacerbate symptoms in susceptible individuals.

Take the case of Diane, who in her early 60s had suffered from abdominal pain, gas, bloating, cramps, and diarrhea on almost a daily basis for years. She also had frequent bouts of sinus infections, requiring antibiotics, and had been diagnosed with rheumatoid arthritis, requiring various immunosuppressive drugs. She was not taking any pharmacological medications when she came to see me because she had very uncomfortable side effects from the immunosuppressive drugs. Her main concerns at the time were frequent, urgent trips to the bathroom, and persistent aching in her hands.

As part of her evaluation, I uncovered an almost addictive passion for milk and dairy products. After explaining the rationale for my recommendation, she reluctantly went on a dairy-free elimination diet for one month. During that time she noticed a significant decrease in the pain in her hands, but only a slight improvement in her IBS symptoms. A lab test for colonic microorganisms showed that the yeast count was very high. Continuing her dairy-free diet, we eliminated dietary refined sugars and yeast-containing foods. She took a six week course of an anti-yeast antibiotic and started supplementation with *Lactobacillus aci-*

dophilus capsules at each meal. When she returned one month later to see me, her hands were pain-free and her IBS symptoms were significantly reduced in terms of their frequency and intensity. Four months later she was free of all IBS symptoms.

Treating Coexisting Conditions

IBS can be categorized by the type of symptoms that predominate: diarrhea, constipation, or a mixture of the two. We can also categorize IBS by the functional changes that occur within and outside of the intestinal tract. Based on these functional changes, specific subsets of treatments can be determined. For example, the individual who has IBS and suffers from fibromyalgia has tender muscle points in various parts of the body. Specific treatment might include magnesium oxide 500 milligrams and malic acid 1200 milligrams twice a day, along with herbal and nutritional measures to calm the bowel.

Another example is the person who suffers from very significant fatigue and IBS. Lab studies might show excessive free radicals, which are the cell-damaging products of metabolic waste. Along with IBS treatment, measures to counteract the free radicals might be vitamin C 1000 milligrams twice a day, vitamin E 800 units a day, alpha lipoic acid 100 milligrams twice a day, and proanthocyanidins 50 milligrams a day.

The Importance of Pure Water

It has been my experience that purified water can play a major role in reducing IBS symptoms for a majority of sufferers. For pure water to have a significant effect, drinking at least 64 ounces per day is a good start. Tap water may be thought of as biologically safe due to the content of an added antiseptic such as chlorine. But in some people, chlorine can act as a direct intestinal irritant, making IBS symptoms worse. One of the best sources of biologically and chemically safe water is from a reverse osmosis filter system, which removes chemical impurities, toxins, and microbes from the water. These systems can be obtained from water purification companies or purchased at health food or hardware stores.

Rhonda's case shows how water filtration eliminated IBS symptoms.

Rhonda moved to Colorado from another state. She had been afflicted by terrible cramps and frequents stools most days of her adult life. She mentioned to me how awful water tasted to her and therefore she drank very little. I advised her to try distilled water from the grocery store for two weeks to see what would happen. When she returned, she reported having gone almost a week without cramps and diarrhea. Then she had a reverse osmosis filter installed in her home and has continued to do well. While it is unusual that water filtration alone cures IBS symptoms, this example shows the importance of pure water.

The Value of Vitamins

I am convinced that in an ideal world, we would obtain all of our vitamin and supplement needs from our food and drink. But in reality, we don't. Many of the foods we eat are already depleted in nutrients by the time they get to our tables. In addition, these foods contain toxins from pesticides and antibiotics and hormones used in meat production. Consequently, we not only need vitamins and supplements, but in some cases much more than the government's recommended daily allowance of nutrients. There are hundreds of vitamins on the market, but for treating IBS, I recommend the following vitamins, at the minimum.

Vitamin C is a strong antioxidant that works on mucous membrane surfaces and in the body's water compartments. IBS patients need to carefully determine what dose they can tolerate. Exceeding tolerance can cause loose stools. A typical dose range is 500 to 2000 milligrams per day. I am reminded of Greg, a 36-year-old salesman who appeared to have all the symptoms of IBS. He was always on the go and frequently missed meals. Instead of eating snacks, he would take a lot of chewable vitamin C. When he came to see me, he complained of gas, cramps, and diarrhea. It turned out that he was consuming ten to twenty 500-milligram chewable vitamin C tablets per day. After eliminating the vitamin and eating several small meals spread out during the day, he became free of his gastrointestinal complaints. After a period of three months, Greg included vitamin C in his diet again, but in a dose he could tolerate without problems.

Vitamin E is essential for the integrity of cellular membranes that line the intestinal tract. It helps to eliminate the adverse effects of free radicals (harmful by-products of toxins and metabolic waste), and also plays a role in the digestion and absorption of fatty foods. A deficiency of this vitamin may result in IBS-like symptoms of intestinal irritability, loose stools, and malabsorption of fats. Dose range is 400 to 800 units of mixed natural tocopherols per day. If the mixed preparation is not available use the d-alpha tocopherol product.

The B-vitamin family is a diverse group of compounds that enter into hundreds of cellular reactions in the body. B vitamin deficiencies may result in diarrhea along with other symptoms. In choosing a B-vitamin preparation, pay particular attention to the doses of B-6, B-12, and folic acid. These three are involved in many critical reactions. All the rest of the B vitamins (thiamine, riboflavin, niacin, pantothenic acid, and biotin) are important and should be included in your vitamin preparation. Vitamin B-6 should be in a range of 50 to 100 milligrams per day. Vitamin B-12 dose is quite variable, with 100 to 500 micrograms being the common therapeutic oral doses; it is also available as sublingual drops and by injection. The usual dose of folic acid is a range of 400 to 800 micrograms. (Note that recent evidence suggests that a folic acid deficiency may be a risk factor for heart attacks.) The dose of the remaining B vitamins is not as critical, and can be taken according to the manufacturer's determination.

TIPS ABOUT VITAMIN C TOLERANCE

Vitamin C, taken in large dosages, can cause GI symptoms that mimic IBS. To determine your own vitamin C tolerance, take 500-milligram increments until GI disturbances develop or worsen. Then reduce your dosage by 500 to 1000 milligram increments. When GI symptoms disappear, you have reached your tolerated dose.

Antioxidants are important adjuncts to vitamin therapy. For example, alpha lipoic acid, a very powerful antioxidant, binds heavy metals in the gut, rendering them less likely to damage intestinal cells. It also helps to regenerate used-up vitamins C and E, enabling them to perform their free-radical scavenger function. The usual dose range of alpha lipoic acid is 100 to 250 milligrams per day. Proanthocyanidins, natural antioxidants derived from grape seeds or pine bark, are very potent and help to clean up an adverse intestinal environment. Their usual dose is 50 to 100 milligrams a day.

Herbal Therapy

Herbs have been used for centuries to treat diseases and disorders, and are still used by most of the world's population. Just as herbs have medicinal properties, they also have side-effects and some people are sensitive or allergic to different ones. An important rule for using herbs is to take them upon prescription by a qualified health practitioner. I have found the following herbs to be effective in treating my patients with IBS.

Peppermint oil is one of the best studied herbs for the treatment of IBS. Used in an enteric-coated form, it bypasses the stomach and is released in the small intestine where it relaxes smooth muscle contractions (that is, relieves cramps). I not only recommend the enteric-coated preparation, which may be difficult to find, but also endorse peppermint tea, which is readily available. Although weaker in strength, the tea is effective for mild cramps. Be sure that the tea preparation has no caffeine added. The standard dose is one to two enteric-coated tabs taken orally three times a day, one to three cups of tea daily.

Fennel oil has been used for centuries as a remedy for IBS symptoms. It has anti-spasmodic effects like peppermint oil. People who are allergic to celery, carrot, or mugwort may have a reaction to fennel oil, as all of these plants are members of the Apiaceae family. The standard daily dose is 0.1 to 0.6 milliliters total, taken orally on food or in a capsule. Do not exceed two weeks of daily use without consulting your doctor because one of its chemical constituents, estragole, can be potentially toxic to the liver. There is an enteric-coated combination that contains peppermint oil and fennel oil, called Pepogest and made by Biotherapies. It can be obtained by special order from your health food store; the usual dose is one tablet, three times a day.

Valerian root also has anti-spasmodic properties and some sedative effects as well. IBS sufferers who have anxiety may find this herb useful.

Because of sedation, it is important to start off with a small dose and gauge its effect before moving on to higher doses. The standard dose is one to three milliliters of the tincture up to three times a day; or dried extract, 450 milligram capsules, one to three times a day.

Cat's claw, which comes from the bark of a tree in Peru, is used worldwide as an intestinal cleanser of intestinal yeast and other pathogenic microorganisms. To make a tea, boil one gram of bark in one cup of water for 15 minutes; cool, strain, and consume three times a day. One to two milliliters of tincture can be taken three times a day. Dried extract, 60-milligram capsules can be taken three times a day.

Deglycyrrhizinated licorice (DGL) is useful in IBS. It helps to stimulate the secretion of and improve the quality of the protective mucous coating on the intestinal cells so that nutrients bind better to the intestinal surfaces. The standard dose is one 200- to 300-milligram tablet or one-half to one teaspoon of tincture before meals and at bedtime.

Ginger root is helpful for an upset stomach and motion sickness. For the treatment of IBS, it may calm the stomach, which may help some patients reduce symptoms of gas and bloating. Like peppermint, ginger may worsen heartburn, so it may be prudent to start with smaller doses. If you have diabetes, heart disease, hypertension, gallbladder disease, or take an anticoagulant, do not take this herb without the advice of your doctor. The standard dose is one to four 250-milligram capsules, three times a day as needed. To make a tea, boil one gram of ginger root in six ounces of water, steep for 15 minutes, then strain and consume three times a day.

Bacteria—Helpful and Harmful

Microorganisms play an important role in health and disease. The intestinal environment is no exception. Identification and elimination of intestinal pathogenic microorganisms may greatly help IBS patients. There are specialized medical laboratories, such as Great Smokies Diagnostic Laboratory, that recover, identify, and quantify the helpful and harmful stool organisms. Armed with this information, the doctor can recommend measures that remove the unwanted ones and replace them with beneficial bacteria. With proper treatment, there can be a significant relief of symptoms.

Although medical science has uncovered a great many viruses, bacteria, yeast, and parasites that cause intestinal difficulties, we must recognize that others have yet to be identified. For example, only recently have we understood that *Helicobacter pylori* can cause stomach ulcers in certain susceptible people, and a course of antibiotics may be curative. In my practice in Colorado, I must keep an eye out for the one-celled organism *Giardia lamblia,* known to cause IBS-like symptoms, but easily eradicated with an antibiotic.

Probiotics are healthy bacteria introduced into the colon that establish and maintain normal bowel function. These bacteria have vital functions for health, including production of natural antimicrobial substances, prevention or improvement of infectious diarrhea, stimulation of immunity, bowel detoxification, and inhibition of certain enzymes associated with GI tract cancers.

In my opinion, every IBS patient should consider taking probiotics because of their positive health potential. If antibiotics are necessary to treat any infection, concurrent use of probiotics for three to six weeks afterward is mandatory. The two most important probiotics are *Lactobacillus acidophilus* and *Bifidobacter.* In the gut, they make up the bulk of the healthy bacterial flora. Probiotic supplementation should include both.

Many brands are available that combine *Lactobacillus* and *Bifidobacter.* I recommend strains of bacteria that are certified to be stomach-acid resistant, such as the NCFM strain. Once past the stomach, these bacteria must adhere to the intestinal cells and be able to multiply. The NCFM strain is probably the most studied in regard to its ability to deliver viable bacteria into the colon. A refrigerated product in a glass jar keeps the bacteria cells from acquiring moisture, which leads to spoilage.

Controversy exists as to the best time to take probiotics. Some say to take them before a meal. Others insist they should be taken with or after a meal. In my opinion, a hearty strain of probiotic culture properly stored can be taken at any time. The usual dose is one to two capsules or one-half teaspoon of the powder with each meal during therapy, or once a day for maintenance.

Digestive Enzymes

Impaired digestion can lead to malabsorption of nutrients thereby causing symptoms of intestinal irritability, gas, bloating, and diarrhea. Proper digestion requires adequate amounts of stomach hydrochloric acid and digestive enzymes, which break down the proteins, fats, and sugars into small, absorbable units. When the stomach does not make enough acid, or the pancreas produces insufficient amounts of its digestive enzymes, then supplementation with digestive enzymes is helpful.

The diagnosis of digestive impairment can be ascertained by a special analysis of the stool, which can be requested by your doctor. The comprehensive digestive stool analysis is one such test that gives detailed information about digestion, absorption, and the microorganisms in the colon. (Physicians can order kits from Great Smokies Diagnostic Laboratory.)

Correction of digestive problems encompasses replacement of any factors that may be low or missing. Betaine hydrochloride can be taken with meals to increase stomach acid. If pancreatic enzyme insufficiency is found, these can be augmented by a prescription of Viokase or any number of over-the-counter, plant-derived, digestive enzyme products at your health food store. Generally, the dose for digestive enzyme replacement is one to three capsules taken at the start of each meal. Another helpful product is BEANO, which breaks down pectin, a compound sugar that results in gas formation in the colon as a result of eating beans or other gas-producing foods such as broccoli and cauliflower. A few drops under the tongue or a tablet or two swallowed at the beginning of a serving can definitely make a meal more agreeable.

Diagnostic Tests

Finally, the patient with IBS who has not responded to any of the above diagnoses and treatments may need in-depth testing. Diagnostic tests are available to identify impaired hepatic detoxification, oxidative

THE CAM APPROACH TO IBS

1. Identification and avoidance of offending foods
2. Aerobic exercise
3. Adequate amounts of pure water
4. A good therapeutic multivitamin
5. Herbal/nutritional/antioxidant support
6. Identification and elimination of intestinal pathogens
7. Replenish the colon with healthy bacteria (probiotics)
8. Further testing and treatment when appropriate

stress, rapid intestinal transit time, and intestinal permeability.

Impaired hepatic detoxification refers to the inability of the detoxification enzymes in the liver and gut to break down toxic metabolic substances that enter the body. In a healthy, fully active system, the toxins are rapidly converted into harmless molecules that are excreted as waste. Defects in one or more key detoxification enzymes can be investigated and weak or missing enzymes can be restored. Toxic substances that remain in the body will eventually do damage to the intestinal cell walls, resulting in IBS-like symptoms or even inflammation. This problem can be helped by supplements that aid in proper detoxification.

Oxidative stress is a term used to describe the overload of free radicals in the body. A free radical is an electrically unstable molecule looking for anything that will react with it. These free radicals are partly the result of normal metabolism, but can be produced with any kind of tissue injury such as radiation, heat, cold, toxins, and infection. When free radicals do damage to intestinal cells, symptoms of abdominal pain, cramps, and diarrhea may result. The diagnosis can be made with an oxidative stress panel. Correction of the underlying cause of free radicals and antioxidant therapy are the mainstays of treatment.

Rapid gut motility, also called rapid intestinal transit time, is a condition in which food leaves the stomach and arrives in the colon much faster than normal. There is reduced absorption of nutrients and increased bacterial gas production in the colon. Cramps and loose, watery, foul-smelling stools may also result. Certain conditions cause a degree of rapid gut transit, including lactase deficiency, food intolerance, and intestinal infections. Treatment is the addition of fiber to the diet and correction of any other underlying conditions.

Increased intestinal permeability or leaky gut syndrome is a condition in which the small intestine allows potentially injurious molecules to pass from the intestinal lumen into the blood. Normally the cells that line the intestine are sandwiched next to one another very tightly. Various conditions that cause damage to these cells or that create swelling between the cells may result in channels for large molecules and infectious agents to gain access into the body. Maldigestion and intestinal infections are two of the more common causes that may result in the leaky gut syndrome. Symptoms include gas, cramping, and diarrhea. Unchecked, this condition may lead to very serious inflammation in the intestines or other organs. Treatment involves looking for the underlying causes and correcting them.

The Natural Way Takes Time

It is worthwhile to learn as much as you can about your intestinal tract. Make the changes in your diet that need to be made. Take the supplements that you and your doctor deem to be most helpful. Above all, be patient! The natural way takes longer for results to be seen. As the bowel becomes more healthy and balanced, your IBS symptoms will decrease. It is my hope that as more evidence-based research becomes available, there will be even more treatments for IBS in the years ahead.

CHAPTER 15

Treating Recurring Symptoms

Tʜᴇ ꜱʏᴍᴘᴛᴏᴍꜱ of IBS are often intermittent and unpredictable. By now, you will have begun to realize that there is no single treatment, trick, or "cure" for the disorder. Many people improve dramatically with dietary and lifestyle changes, and with stress reduction. However, they may have one or two lingering symptoms that become a constant or recurring source of aggravation.

Dealing with Lingering Symptoms

Luc is a 37-year-old real estate professional, working in a crowded real estate office. In many ways, Luc was a classic IBS patient. He had suffered from cramping abdominal pain and irregular bowel movements. He also complained of belching, bloating, and excessive gas. After I had concluded that we were dealing with IBS, I outlined a program of specific treatment recommendations. He responded well to the treatment plan but continued to experience gas.

"Doc," he confided, "I pass enough gas in an afternoon to fill a hot-air balloon. It's embarrassing and uncomfortable, and I can't always control it. I'm afraid that if you can't help me with this problem, my coworkers may see to it that I'm exiled to a deserted island." Then with a grin he added, "It's a good thing it's a nonsmoking office, because there are times it would definitely be inadvisable to light up."

In order of importance, the goals of IBS therapy consist of regularizing the bowel movements and relieving abdominal pain. If you are able to develop a consistent pattern of bowel movements that are neither too hard nor too soft, the abdominal pain will often, in turn, be relieved. Your other symptoms, such as bloating and gas, will also improve once you establish regular, consistent bowel movements. As you know, the pain of an IBS attack is usually relieved by a bowel movement, and that bloated feeling is lessened if you are not constipated.

Luc simply got carried away with the recommendation of increased dietary fiber. As many do, he thought that if some fiber is good, more will be better. After this was brought to his attention, he decreased his daily intake of fiber and has continued to do well.

Increasing Dietary Fiber

As outlined in Chapter 6, gradually increasing dietary fiber is an excellent way to regularize bowel movements. Fiber is the undigested portion of complex carbohydrates (grains, fruits, vegetables, beans), which remains in the intestinal tract to exert a beneficial effect. Fiber will add bulk to the stool, making a hard stool softer and a soft stool more firm. The addition of fiber will be most beneficial for the sufferers with constipation and a hard stool. Fiber supplements may be added to your diet if you cannot maintain an adequate fiber intake by increasing the amount of complex carbohydrates you eat.

If you do take fiber supplements, be sure to take them around mealtime so that they can mix well with the food. For some reason, many people get into a habit of taking their fiber supplements at night, just before retiring. This is not the best time, and you may end up with a hard stool lodged in the bowel and a gelatinous mass (the fiber) attempting to push it out. If you take the fiber supplement at mealtime, it will mix with the food, providing for a consistent, moist, bulky stool.

TIP about Dietary Fiber to Relieve Diarrhea: Although once considered helpful for diarrhea, increasing dietary fiber or adding fiber supplements to your diet has not been found to lessen the discomfort associated with diarrhea.

Achieving Regularity

"How often should I have a bowel movement?" is a question I am frequently asked. Most medical authorities contend that "normal" bowel function varies between three bowel movements a day and three bowel movements a week. These estimates imply that if you have more than three bowel movements a day, you have diarrhea, and if you have fewer than three a week, you are constipated. However, this so-called normal range has been established on the observation that the majority of people in the western world fall between these two extremes. Realize that what is normal for you may not be an optimal frequency of bowel movements for someone else. Furthermore, the frequency of your bowel movements may not be as important as the consistency of the stool. You may have a daily bowel movement that is very hard and difficult to pass, suggesting constipation. Conversely, you may have rather infrequent bowel movements that are loose and watery when they occur, suggesting diarrhea.

TIPS ON NORMAL BOWEL FUNCTION

The frequency of your bowel movements may not be as important as the consistency of the stools. Stools should be neither too hard nor too loose. The passage of stool should not be associated with cramps, bloating, or discomfort.

Although regular bowel movements are important in helping to relieve IBS symptoms, it is also important not to become insistent on this fact. The fact that you do not have a bowel movement does not necessarily point to a problem unless you experience pain, discomfort, and bloating because you have not had a bowel movement.

The Outhouse Theory

There are several likely explanations for the apparent increase in IBS and other bowel problems in recent years. I propose what I have come to refer to as the outhouse theory. Persons living in rural areas in the past ate a much more balanced, wholesome diet than we tend to eat today in our urbanized, fast-paced society. In addition, in the days before modern rest rooms, the outhouse was the temple of elimination. Many of my older patients who grew up during this era become quite distressed when there is a change in their "regularity" (a valid concern, since this may be a warning signal of colon cancer). These patients tell me that for as long as they can remember, they have had regular bowel movements. They recall scheduled early-morning treks to the outhouse to relieve themselves, before they left the house to start their day.

In today's society, we take for granted the fact that toilets are readily accessible. There is no need to plan a certain time for elimination. ("I will go when I get the urge, whether at home, at work, or in a public facility.") This approach leads to a problem with timing. It may not be convenient for you to go when the need arises, since you may be in an important business meeting or stuck in traffic. And after "holding it" for a period of time, the urge will often lessen to the point where you no longer feel the need. This both conscious and subconscious blocking of impulses from the rectum may ultimately lead to constipation. You may later experience uncomfortable cramps, and then, when you have to go, you have to go!

How to Prevent Constipation

You can begin to see that one of the most important ways to avoid constipation is to establish a consistent time for elimination. This is what I refer to as "adult toilet training." For most, the best time is after breakfast. The fact is, meals stimulate the gastrocolic reflex and may facilitate a bowel movement after, for example, a bowl of cereal. As food enters the stomach, a series of events that facilitate digestion is set into motion. The hormone cholecystokinin is released; in addition to stimulating gallbladder contractions, it also stimulates colon contractions—leading to defecation. This hormone is believed to mediate the gastro-(stomach) colic (colon) reflex, which is exaggerated in some IBS sufferers.

Many patients tell me they are not hungry early in the morning. This is no doubt true, as their systems have been conditioned to skip breakfast, much as an infant may be conditioned to feed on a regular schedule. Perhaps you are the type of person who likes to sleep as long as possible. Since you know it takes exactly 24 minutes to commute to your job, you set the alarm for 7:12 a.m. so that you can be dressed and out of the house by 7:34 a.m. This leaves you precisely two minutes to spare before beginning work at 8:00 a.m. And breakfast consists of coffee and doughnuts in the office during your first break at 10:15 a.m.

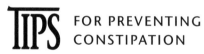 **FOR PREVENTING CONSTIPATION**

- Increase dietary fiber.
- Establish a routine time and place for elimination.
- Allow adequate time for a bowel movement.
- Regular exercise may help prevent constipation.
- Do not habitually use laxatives. (Fiber supplements, however, are not laxatives in the true sense of the word and may be safely used.)
- If you do take laxatives (whether prescription or over-the-counter), use them only for a short period of time, and only under direction of a physician.

Why not try taking a break when you first arise? Set the alarm for 6:45 a.m. and use the extra time to eat a balanced, wholesome breakfast at home and to have a bowel movement. This will help relieve your stress level too, since rushing to work tends to set the pace for the remainder of your day.

What about enemas? Like laxative abuse, the abuse or overuse of enemas may cause problems in the long run because your rectum can become dependent on this procedure. However, an occasional enema may be an effective way to stimulate a bowel movement "from below." And this technique may provide the most immediate relief from the pain and bloating associated with constipation.

How to Prevent Diarrhea

If you suffer from IBS and have a tendency towards diarrhea, look closely for triggers. I find that diarrhea-predominant IBS patients have food intolerance or allergies more frequently than their constipation-predominant counterparts. A study published in the journal *Gut* suggests that food intolerances are more common in patients who first complain of gas. The most common foods to trigger an episode include dairy products, sweets, and fatty foods. Refer to Chapter 4, "What You Should Know About Diet," for a more detailed explanation of dietary triggers.

Remember that the mechanisms underlying food intolerance are complex, and do not be too quick to eliminate certain foods from your diet without first consulting a physician. Too often I have seen patients who have placed themselves needlessly on very restrictive diets as a result of inconclusive analysis. In these cases further investigation revealed that the list of foods causing a problem was much shorter than previously suspected.

Emotional stress is a frequent cause of so-called nervous diarrhea. If stress triggers diarrhea in your case, refer to Chapter 9, "Stress and the Intestinal Tract." Learn, practice, and experiment with different stress reduction techniques to alleviate stress-induced diarrhea. If these measures fail, your doctor may recommend various medications to treat symptomatic diarrhea. These medications are most useful on a short-term, as-needed basis, such as when you are traveling, or where bathrooms are not readily accessible. Take care to not overdo it, or you will end up constipated. Keep in mind that peppermint is an anti-spasmodic that may relieve diarrhea and associated cramps. I have many patients who find caffeine-free peppermint tea very calming to the gut.

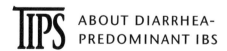

TIPS ABOUT DIARRHEA-PREDOMINANT IBS

Generally speaking, avoid dairy products, foods with high fat content, and sugar.

How to Prevent Abdominal Pain

Your stress reduction techniques and peppermint tea can also be helpful when you are experiencing abdominal pain and cramps. Try relaxing when the urge to defecate or expel gas occurs; this could alleviate symptoms.

Some of my patients find a brisk walk helps to reduce the spasms, and this might also facilitate the passage of gas. Others have said that a warm bath seems to help.

Try focusing your attention on something—anything—other than the pain. With time, the painful spasms will usually pass. Only if all these measures have failed, try taking the anti-spasmodic medication your doctor may have prescribed.

How to Prevent Excessive Gas

If you have a problem with gas, you need not feel alone. The production and passage of gas is normal, although many consider it socially unacceptable. The source of many a joke, it can be an embarrassing, uncomfortable, and continual problem.

The symptoms of excessive gas may consist of belching (eructation), bloating, abdominal pain, and passing gas from the colon (flatus). How is excessive gas defined? Well, believe it or not, the technology is available to measure daily gas production, and studies have been done. The data seem to suggest that IBS sufferers do not produce excessive amounts of gas in comparison with people without IBS. Rather, IBS patients are more sensitive to normal amounts of gas present in the intestinal tract.

The majority of gas in the intestinal tract comes from swallowed air. Also, anything that increases the production of saliva will contribute to increased air swallowing (aerophagia). Part of the "fight or flight" stress response is increased salivation, and nervous tension may therefore be a factor. Cigarette smoking and the use of gum and mints also increases salivation and air swallowing. The ingestion of carbonated beverages contributes to intestinal gas. Perhaps you recall the time you quickly downed a pop or beer. You felt bloated, and may have felt better after you burped. If the gas does not exit upwards, it will eventually find its way out the other direction. Air swallowing may lead to excessive accumulation of gas in the stomach, which may produce a bloated feeling and pain in the upper abdomen. Belching often makes this condition better.

A word of caution is in order here. There is a difference between a spontaneous belch and a forced belch. A spontaneous belch occurs when air trapped in the stomach escapes through the esophagus, resulting in lessened pressure and decreased bloating. Having observed this, many people attempt to make themselves belch when they feel bloated. However, it has been shown that forced belching is accomplished by actually swallowing air and then belching it back up. More often than not, more air is swallowed than is brought back up by forced belching. The net effect is one of worsening symptoms, since a perpetual cycle develops in which more air accumulates in the stomach. Some people drink

TIPS ON DECREASING INTESTINAL GAS

- At mealtime, eat slowly and chew your food well in a relaxed environment.
- Avoid excessive liquids at mealtime. Do not "wash down" your food.
- Avoid carbonated beverages.
- Avoid using chewing gum, mints, and tobacco products, which all increase air swallowing.
- Try to determine which foods in your diet are easily digested.
- If you are in the process of adding fiber to your diet, do so slowly, allowing your intestinal tract time to adjust.
- Wear comfortable, loose clothing.

carbonated beverages to facilitate belching and relieve the bloated feeling. This practice may ultimately worsen the symptoms associated with air swallowing.

Air in the stomach that is not released by belching will pass along with the chyme into the small intestine, then the large intestine, and eventually out of the rectum as flatus. Along this route, pockets of air may become trapped, producing bloating and "gas pains."

As air rises, it will have the tendency to accumulate in the uppermost areas of the intestine. Two such areas are the upper right colon (hepatic flexure) and the upper left colon (splenic flexure).

Some people have a predisposition to the trapping of air in one or the other area, producing bloating and pain, referred to as either the hepatic or splenic flexure syndrome. The more common splenic flexure syndrome may produce pain that radiates from the left upper abdomen to the left shoulder area.

The discomfort of gas pains may mimic a heart attack. Since heart disease is much more common than splenic flexure syndrome, be sure to consult your physician if you experience this type of discomfort.

In addition to swallowed air, the digestion and fermentation of certain foods will produce intestinal gas. As explained earlier, complex carbohydrates, particularly those with a high water-soluble fiber content such as beans, are the greatest gas producers. There does seem to be individual variation in how much gas is produced with certain foods. This variation may be related to varying degrees of carbohydrate malabsorption, such as that seen with lactose intolerance. Lactose intolerance is not an all-or-none phenomenon. There appears to be a certain threshold above which the lactose load exceeds the body's ability to break down the lactose. A half cup of milk may be tolerated, whereas a whole cup of milk will produce gas in the same person. You may need to do some detective work to determine what foods may be contributing to excessive gas in your case. Your diet diary would be a helpful tool for this endeavor.

CHAPTER 16

Facts About
Coexisting Conditions

IBS, PMS, FMS—sounds a little like some sort of alphabet soup, doesn't it?

Helen, who works as a grocery store cashier, is a good example of someone with this combination of problems. On her first visit, she proclaimed, "I feel like a hypochondriac." She said she had been having problems with her bowels for most of her life. The cramps and diarrhea usually worsened, however, 7 to 10 days before the onset of her menstrual flow. She suspected, after reading a magazine article, that she had PMS (premenstrual syndrome). In addition to her bowel complaints, she experienced mood swings, breast tenderness, and fluid retention during the premenstrual phase. Over the past few years, she had come to accept these symptoms as her fate. Only after she began to experience extreme fatigue and generalized aches did she decide to seek medical attention.

After preliminary evaluation, I determined that Helen had developed, over the preceding 12 months, symptoms consistent with the diagnosis of FMS (fibromyalgia syndrome), in addition to her symptoms of IBS and PMS. FMS, previously referred to as fibrositis, is a common disorder affecting an estimated three to six million people in the United States.

FMS, like IBS, occurs more frequently in women than in men, and of course PMS occurs only in women (although some women contend that men go through similar cyclic changes). It is uncommon for all three disorders to be present and create a significant problem in one person, as they did with Helen. It is not uncommon, however, for two of these three problems to coexist.

PMS

Up to 90 percent of women admit to having some form of premenstrual discomfort. The majority of these women experience mild symptoms that do not interfere with normal daily activities. The lifestyle and dietary changes recommended to treat PMS are similar to those recommended to control IBS symptoms, so if you suffer from both problems, you should be able to improve both conditions simultaneously by following the guidelines in this book.

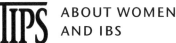 **ABOUT WOMEN AND IBS**

In North America, IBS affects predominately females. According to a U.S. national survey completed in 1999, compared with the general population, women with IBS:

• Have three times as many sick days
• Are twice as likely to limit the kind or amount of work they do
• Must limit other activities, such as social activities and travel.

Symptoms of PMS

The symptoms of PMS vary greatly among individuals. In addition, the number and magnitude of symptoms associated with PMS may vary with each cycle or at different stages of life for each person. Although the symptoms of PMS could well fill a text, these are the more common, generally accepted symptoms: mood swings (anxiety, depression), irritability, headaches, breast swelling and tenderness, menstrual cramps, fluid retention, fatigue, and cravings for certain foods (especially sweets).

The hallmark of the disorder is the occurrence of these symptoms 10 to 14 days before the onset of the menstrual flow—hence the name premenstrual syndrome. Studies show that the number of psychiatric admissions, accidents, and suicide attempts among women increases during the premenstrual phase. This phenomenon indicates that mood changes can be quite severe.

Many IBS patients report worsening IBS symptoms in their premenstrual phase. These symptoms may be the result of hormonal changes that occur during the menstrual cycle, or they might occur as the result of eating salty foods, sweets, and other foods that PMS sufferers tend to crave.

A study reported in *Gastroenterology* found that 34 percent of 233 planned parenthood clients who denied symptoms of IBS reported that menstruation was associated with one or more bowel symptoms. IBS patients from the gastroenterology clinic were significantly more likely to experience worsening bowel symptoms, especially increased gas, during menses. It appears that bowel dysfunction increases during the menstrual flow in PMS patients with and without established IBS.

TIPS ABOUT ILLNESS AND WOMEN WITH IBS

The U.S. 1999 national survey also reported that women with IBS had 71 percent more abdominal or intestinal surgeries than women without IBS. The survey also found a much higher rate of illness among women with IBS. A history of abuse and severe IBS has been linked to increased use of medical treatments and unnecessary procedures. Also, women in North America may deal with psychological distress by developing or seeking relief from physical illness, while men under stress have been socialized to express their anger.

Diagnosis and Treatment of PMS

Although PMS was described more than 50 years ago, there is no general consensus as to the cause or treatment. Nor is there a specific test to diagnose PMS. As with IBS, the diagnosis is suggested by the patient's history, and the physical exam and any tests are used to exclude other disorders, such as endometriosis and ovarian cysts.

Therapy for PMS focuses on education, exercise, and diet. (Sound familiar?) It is important to realize that PMS is a common problem; it is not all in your head, and you are not just "going crazy." The education process begins with learning what is and what is not known about PMS. Current theories suggest a relationship between hormonal imbalances and PMS symptoms. However, the exact underlying abnormalities are not fully understood.

Exercise is of immediate benefit by providing an outlet for pent-up tension. Regular exercise also lessens fatigue as physical endurance increases.

The PMS prevention diet is similar to the "ideal diet" outlined in Chapter 4, "What You Should Know About Diet." This diet emphasizes whole, fresh foods, frequent small feedings, and avoiding caffeine, sugar, fat, and processed foods. I have found the craving for sweets seems to worsen the mood swings, which may be the result of erratic fluctuations in blood glucose. One tip is that chromium supplements, easily obtained at health food stores, may help to smooth out these wide glucose fluctuations and curb the craving for sweets. Eating too many sweets may also cause abdominal bloating and excessive gas, and increased salt intake invariably worsens premenstrual fluid retention. Caffeine has been implicated as a factor in breast swelling and tenderness in fibrocystic breast disease.

As part of the treatment of PMS, your physician may request that you keep a "menstrual diary" to record symptoms, daily weight, and the onset of menses. This diary may be kept in conjunction with a diet diary. The purpose of the menstrual diary is to characterize your symptoms (such as mood changes, irritability, breast swelling, and menstrual cramps) and to determine whether there is a consistent relationship between these symptoms and the menstrual cycle.

Some investigators believe that vitamin E and vitamin B6 may help, particularly with regard to breast swelling and tenderness. Check with your physician regarding the proper dosages, since excessive amounts of vitamin B6 may cause nerve damage. Various other vitamin and mineral supplements have been marketed in recent years for treatment of PMS. Your physician may discuss the various pharmacologic treatment modalities with you if "first-line therapy" is ineffective.

FMS

Fibromyalgia syndrome is one of the more common conditions encountered in medical practice. It belongs to the family of rheumatic diseases, which affect the joints, tendons, muscles, and ligaments. Various types of arthritis, bursitis, and tendonitis are common examples of diseases that fall into the specialty of rheumatology. Although a common cause of chronic pain and fatigue, FMS fortunately is not a degenerative, deforming process, and it is not life-threatening.

Although no direct association has been firmly established between FMS and IBS, irritable bowel symptoms are one of the diagnostic criteria considered for the diagnosis of fibromyalgia, suggesting a possible relationship.

Dr. Don Goldenberg reported in the Journal of the American Medical Association *(JAMA)*: "Since fibromyalgia shares many common features with other poorly described, chronic pain conditions, including…irritable bowel syndrome, each of these disorders should be evaluated in similar pathophysiologic fashion and compared with fibromyalgia." Another study, from the British *Journal of Rheumatology*, indicated that 70 percent of FMS patients had IBS and 65 percent of IBS patients had FMS.

Symptoms of FMS

The prominent feature of FMS is a generalized deep muscular aching discomfort in the absence of other conditions to account for these symptoms. It is similar to having a tension headache of the entire body. Although the discomfort is not always generalized, there are common so-called trigger points where you may note tenderness with firm pressure. These trigger points include the area between the neck and shoulders, where the knees would touch if you put them together, the back, the chest, and the buttocks. These symptoms often occur in association with headaches, disturbed sleep, morning stiffness, and fatigue.

Causes and Treatment of FMS

Although the exact cause of FMS is unknown and there is no specific test to establish the diagnosis, it may occur in association with another established rheumatic disease, such as rheumatoid arthritis. When that happens, it is referred to as secondary fibromyalgia syndrome because it occurs secondarily to an underlying condition. Symptoms of FMS may develop or worsen after an injury. In the majority of cases, symptoms simply develop and there is no associated rheumatologic disease or inciting event.

Some researchers have postulated that an underlying sleep disorder is the cause of FMS. These researchers found characteristic brain wave patterns in FMS patients during sleep. These patients lacked stage four sleep, which is the so-called restorative phase of sleep. Normal sleep patterns may be broadly divided into rapid eye movement (REM) and non-rapid eye movement (NREM) sleep stages. NREM sleep is divided into four successively deeper stages, with stage four being the deepest. FMS patients reported no difficulty falling asleep and had mostly uninterrupted sleep, but did not feel rested upon awakening. Normal, healthy subjects who were deprived of stage four sleep developed symptoms of FMS, again suggesting a possible association.

This abnormal sleep disturbance, as seen in FMS, has been described in up to 30 percent of IBS patients. In another study published in *Gastroenterology*, IBS sufferers and healthy subjects were examined during wake and sleep. IBS sufferers spent 36 percent of their total sleep time in the REM stage, whereas healthy subjects spent only 18 percent of their total sleep in REM. Dreaming takes place during REM sleep, so if you dream a lot, this may be another sign that you are not getting enough restorative sleep.

Other possible causes of FMS include anxiety and depression, poor posture, and the normal wear and tear of aging. "Stress," which includes tension, anxiety, depression, and pent-up frustrations, will often lead to muscular aching and fatigue.

Antidepressant medications, usually in much lower doses than those employed in treating depression, are very effective for the

TIPS ABOUT SLEEP HYGIENE

Feeling tired day after day from lack of restorative sleep can not only slow your recovery from IBS, but add more stress to your life. To improve your sleep:
- Exercise regularly and add a 20-minute walk after your evening meal.
- Avoid caffeine, especially within six hours before bedtime.
- Don't drink alcohol within several hours of bedtime.
- Don't nap close to bedtime; if you do nap, do so at the same time daily.
- Make your bedroom conducive to sleep by eliminating noise, light, and temperature extremes.
- Establish a regular sleep time.
- Wind down for about 30 minutes before you sleep by reading or bathing.

If these suggestions fail to improve your sleep, try relaxation techniques, biofeedback training, or cognitive behavioral therapy.

treatment of FMS. These medications are believed to exert a beneficial effect on the disordered sleep pattern. They are most helpful if used in combination with an exercise program that increases flexibility and tone, along with some stress reduction techniques. I often use low-dose antidepressant medication as first-line pharmacologic treatment in patients with IBS who also have symptoms suggestive of FMS after they fail to improve with recommended dietary and lifestyle changes. Often a break in the cycle of insomnia-fatigue-insomnia will bring lasting benefit. In less severe cases of insomnia, improved sleep hygiene, stretching exercises, and relaxation techniques are all that is needed.

The Team Approach

With multiple symptoms, you may have to decide whether a primary-care physician or a specialist is the better choice for treatment. The perspective of a primary-care physician (a general internal medicine specialist or family physician) is often different from that of a gastroenterologist. Whereas the gastroenterologist specializes in depth (within the field of gastroenterology), the primary-care physician specializes in breadth (attempting to remain current in all areas of medicine). The primary-care physician may be in a better position to recommend treatments that would, in essence, potentially correct two problems that fall within two separate specialties of medicine. For example, gastroenterologists have special training and expertise in treating IBS, and rheumatologists have special training and expertise in treating FMS. A primary-care physician may know something about both of these disorders and thus may be the best choice for treating someone who suffers from both IBS and FMS.

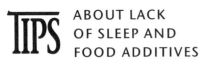

TIPS ABOUT LACK OF SLEEP AND FOOD ADDITIVES

MSG and aspartame may contribute to sleepless nights. Remember that their main ingredients, glutamic acid and aspartic acid respectively, are neuro-excitatory amino acids that may stimulate nerves in the brain in susceptible individuals. So avoid these additives in particular if you have IBS and coexisting symptoms.

With difficult cases, particularly where multiple medical problems that cross specialty designations exist, a coordinated, complementary team approach involving a primary-care physician and a specialist is often the best avenue to proper diagnosis and treatment. Many insurance companies and HMOS (health maintenance organizations) recognize this fact and now require the primary-care physician to coordinate all care given to an individual.

Other Coexisting Conditions

Mixed anxiety and depression (MAD) and generalized anxiety disorder (GAD) are psychological syndromes that often coexist with IBS. By addressing and treating the underlying anxiety or depression as discussed in Chapter 11, IBS symptoms often improve. Counseling and/or medications should be considered early in the course of treatment where these conditions are also present. Remember that a common-sense approach consisting of proper diet, exercise, and stress reduction is often all that is necessary to have a profound positive impact on both IBS and the conditions that coexist with it.

CHAPTER 17

Other Common Gastrointestinal Disorders

T HIS CHAPTER LOOKS at some of the other common disorders of the gastrointestinal tract, not because you are likely to develop any of these other problems, but rather, as the saying goes, because "common things occur commonly," and these conditions may mimic or coexist with IBS.

Many of my patients, for example, have a hiatal hernia as well as IBS. Approximately 20 percent of the population has hiatal hernia. I am frequently asked questions such as: "The upper GI showed a hiatal hernia—is this the cause of my problem?" and "How is IBS different?"

Hemorrhoids are another very common problem that in my experience does seem to be more prevalent in IBS patients. The reason may be that diarrhea and constipation aggravate "piles." Since I frequently counsel patients on how to deal with this "pain in the butt," a word about hemorrhoids is appropriate in a book on IBS.

Our review begins at the upper end of the gastrointesinal tract and works down to the rectum. Then the gallbladder is reviewed, and finally a common infection of the gastrointestinal tract is discussed. This chapter is not an all-inclusive review of every condition that affects the gastrointestinal system but is intended to take some of the mystery out of the common medical problems that affect your gut.

IBS Later in Life

Before we begin our discussion of other common gastrointestinal disorders a word about IBS symptoms in later life may be helpful. As symptoms of IBS usually present themselves earlier in life, the occurrence of IBS symptoms in the elderly is often underappreciated. Functional bowel disorders, including IBS, remain the most common cause of intestinal complaints in people over age 65. As our population ages, physicians can expect to see and treat larger numbers of geriatric patients with IBS.

Symptoms of IBS in the elderly are the same as those seen in younger groups. However, as people age they are more likely to develop other coexisting medical conditions, such as diverticulosis, which occurs in 50 percent of people over age 70. Additionally, the likelihood of developing colon polyps and colon cancer increases with age. If you are an IBS sufferer and have any change in your symptoms—consult your physician! This change in symptoms may represent the development of a more serious, life-threatening condition such as colon cancer. Elderly IBS sufferers who develop gastrointestinal symptoms for the first time will require a more thorough evaluation by their physician.

TIPS ABOUT IBS AND GI DISORDERS

An IBS sufferer is no more likely to develop colon cancer, colitis, or polyps than anyone else. However, having IBS does not protect you from colon cancer or any other common gastrointestinal malady.

Reflux Esophagitis

Did you know that heartburn has nothing to do with your heart? Terms such as "heartburn" and "indigestion" mean different things to different people. For some, "heartburn" refers to that uncomfortable feeling you may experience when you eat too much or too fast. For others, heartburn is an intense burning pain in the upper abdomen and mid-chest that may be associated with a sour taste in the mouth. Physicians technically refer to this condition as reflux esophagitis.

CAUSES AND DIAGNOSIS

As the name implies, the acid contents of the stomach flow back into the esophagus, leading, over time, to inflammation of the esophagus, which in turn leads to esophagitis. Eating too much or too fast may predispose some people to an occasional bout of "acid indigestion." For others, this is a chronic and recurring problem.

A circular ring of muscle divides the lower esophagus from the stomach. This ring, referred to as the lower esophageal sphincter (LES), normally remains contracted and prevents the acid contents of the stomach from moving upward into the esophagus. The swallowing mechanism allows for relaxation of the LES during swallowing. However, if the LES relaxes at other times, regurgitation may occur and heartburn results.

The diagnosis of reflux esophagitis is suggested by the symptoms. X rays of the upper gastrointestinal tract or direct observation through endoscopy help confirm the diagnosis.

TREATMENT

Several general recommendations are often helpful in reducing the frequency and severity of reflux esophagitis symptoms. For obese patients, losing weight tends to reduce abdominal pressure. At the same time, these patients should avoid tight-fitting garments or any activities that increase abdominal pressure. Elevating the head of the bed six to eight inches by placing blocks under the bedpost or frame allows gravity to work for you at night. Sufferers should also avoid stooping or bending shortly after a meal, since these movements encourage reflux into the esophagus.

Foods to avoid include fatty foods, chocolates, alcohol, citrus fruit juices, and coffee. Nicotine in any form, but especially cigarettes, decreases LES tone and should be avoided. Avoid late-night snacks, heavy meals, or lying down shortly after meals. Antacids, which neutralize acid in the esophagus and stomach, are helpful. Take these on an as-needed basis; they usually provide immediate relief. Medications designed to increase LES tone and promote emptying of the stomach may be used alone or in combination with acid-blocking medications to treat reflux esophagitis. Your doctor may also prescribe medications designed to block acid secretion in the stomach. In rare instances, surgery may be required to treat resistant cases.

If the problem is allowed to continue untreated, the esophagus may eventually scar and develop a stricture. Repeated acid irritation of the esophagus may also predispose the sufferer to cancer of the esophagus. This very serious disorder led to John Wayne's death. If you experience difficulty in swallowing or the sensation that food is getting stuck as it goes down, see your physician immediately; these symptoms may indicate stricture formation or esophageal cancer.

COEXISTENCE WITH HIATAL HERNIA

Reflux esophagitis may be associated with a hiatal hernia, the protrusion of a portion of the stomach through the diaphragm into the chest. I have heard patients refer to this common problem as their "high hernia." Hiatal hernias become more common with aging and can occur in up to 70 percent of those over age 60. Most hiatal hernias produce no symptoms, and no treatment is required.

If a patient with reflux has a hiatal hernia, the treatment is the same as for a patient with reflux who does not have a hiatal hernia. Patients with hiatal hernias seem to complain more of bloating after meals and are more likely to experience the relatively uncommon problem of esophageal spasm. When asked what it felt like, one of my patients with this disorder explained: "It is like a charley horse in the center of my chest."

Peptic Ulcer Disease

Unlike the esophagus, which is damaged by acid, the stomach is designed to tolerate, under normal circumstances, the acid produced by specialized cells within the stomach. Peptic ulcers are raw areas that develop either in the stomach (gastric ulcers) or the first part of the small intestine (duodenal ulcers). These raw areas are similar to the mouth ulcers or "canker sores" that many people experience at some time.

SYMPTOMS AND CAUSES

As the stomach acid infiltrates the raw area, an intense, burning pain may be felt, usually just below the breastbone. It is like pouring salt on an open wound. Most, but not all, ulcers produce symptoms that are variously described as "gnawing pains" and "hunger pains." The term "hunger pain" probably arises from the observation that eating food or drinking milk will often temporarily relieve symptoms. The food or milk simply coats the stomach and neutralizes the acid. Although the ingestion of milk provides temporary relief, in the long run excessive milk intake may worsen ulcer symptoms as the calcium in milk encourages increased acid secretion by the stomach.

Ulcer pain frequently occurs at night when the stomach is empty. This is in contrast to the pain of IBS, which experts contend should rarely, if ever, awaken a patient from sleep.

What causes peptic ulcers? The answer to this question has been debated for some time. Under ordinary circumstances there is a balance between appropriate acid production and the stomach lining's defensive mucosal protection against self-digestion by the acid produced. The scale can be tipped by an excess of acid production or a breakdown in the mucosal barrier. What factors upset this delicate balance?

A major breakthrough in the study of ulcer disease was initially described in 1982 by an Australian physician, Dr. Barry Marshall, when he reported a possible association between the bacteria *Helicobacter pylorus*, and the development of ulcer disease and gastritis. His theory was initially met with overwhelming skepticism. To date numerous studies throughout the world have shown a consistently strong association among infection with *H. pylori*, inflammation of the stomach, and ulcer disease. The most convincing evidence comes from studies looking at ulcer recurrence rates in patients given antibiotics to eradicate *H. pylori*.

Emotional stress and smoking may lead to excessive acid production and result in peptic ulcers. Breakdown in the mucosal barriers may occur as a result of taking an anti-inflammatory medication used to treat arthritis and pain. Examples include over-the-counter products such as aspirin, in addition to many prescription medications collectively referred to as NSAIDs (non-steroidal anti-inflammatory drugs).

TREATMENT

Bland diets are no longer recommended for patients with ulcer disease. I tell my patients to avoid only those foods that seem to aggravate symptoms. With many patients, the avoidance of very hot or very spicy foods is all that is necessary as an "ulcer diet."

Physicians continue to treat peptic ulcers with conventional therapy consisting of antacids to neutralize stomach acid, medications designed to decrease acid production, or medications that assist the mucosal defense barriers. Tests are available now to detect the presence of *H. pylori* and antibiotics are added if *H. pylori* is present. Addition of an antibiotic regimen offers the greatest hope for a long-term cure.

SIMILAR CONDITIONS

Some patients have upper abdominal discomfort characterized as burning or bloating that is suggestive of peptic ulcers, but no ulcer is evident by X ray or endoscopy. Physicians believe that these patients have so-called nonulcer dyspepsia or functional dyspepsia. These patients may have low-grade inflammation of the stomach or duodenum, which responds to acid-blocking medication. Alternatively, they may have a disorder of stomach motility.

Intestinal Adhesions

As partially digested food, referred to as chyme, exits the stomach, it enters the small intestine. The small intestine is where the problem of adhesions usually occurs. Adhesions are abnormal fibrous bands or scars that develop between internal organs. Often these bands form between contiguous loops of small intestine, causing the loops to stick together. If you were to observe a surgeon perform a laparotomy (surgery of the abdominal cavity) under ordinary circumstances, you would note the surgeon freely move around or shift the 21 feet of small intestine. Were that same surgeon operating on a patient with adhesions, you would notice that certain portions of the intestine adhere to one another. The significance of adhesions is that they may interfere with the normal peristaltic activity of the small intestine, the rhythmic contractions that move the chyme through the intestine. Interruption of these contractions can lead to intermittent abdominal pain. In some cases, the intestine can become kinked, resulting in an intestinal obstruction.

CAUSES AND DIAGNOSIS

Adhesions most commonly occur some time after a surgical operation. Just as visible scars form on the abdomen during the healing process, scars may form internally as healing progresses. Infections or inflammation of the abdominal cavity increase the likelihood that adhesions will form. For example, surgery for a ruptured appendix, wherein infected material has infiltrated the abdominal cavity, is much more likely to produce adhesions than an appendectomy performed before rupture occurs.

Unfortunately, there is no simple way to determine if adhesions are present without direct visual observation through a laparoscope or during exploratory surgery. And the presence of adhesions is not proof positive they are causing the problem. An upper GI series with small-bowel follow-through may occasionally be helpful in making this determination. I have seen IBS symptoms worsen in numerous patients after an abdominal operation for an unrelated condition. I theorize that in these patients fibrous adhesions of the small intestine may be a cofactor that further interferes with intestinal motility and contributes to worsening symptoms.

TREATMENT

Exploratory or laparoscopic surgery is the only effective treatment for adhesions. Cutting through the adhesive bands may eliminate the problem. Unfortunately, since surgery causes adhesions, there is always risk of recurrence later.

Spigelian Hernia

Spigelian hernias are not really a gastrointestinal disorder, but occur as a result of a protrusion of the intestinal contents through a weak area in the lower lateral abdominal wall. I have found this condition to be more common than the medical literature suggests, as I am often asked to provide a second opinion about patients with vague abdominal pains. At the same time, it is difficult to diagnose; one surgeon reported he was able to secure diagnosis before surgery in only 50 percent of his cases.

The key to diagnosis is recurrent pain and tenderness localized within the abdominal wall. A bulge may be noted, particularly when standing and straining. Symptoms may simulate an intra-abdominal condition, and I have seen patients unfortunately misdiagnosed as having IBS since no other cause for their recurrent pain could be identified.

One factor that predisposes one to the development of spigelian hernia is an abdominal incision, particularly a transverse lower abdominal incision made at the time of a caesarean delivery. Treatment for spigelian hernia is surgical repair.

Diverticulosis/Diverticulitis

Undigested material from the small intestine is propelled forward into the colon or large intestine. It is in the colon where diverticulosis, or the appearance of small outpouchings called diverticula, occurs. The condition becomes more common as people age. Whereas half the population over age 60 has diverticula, they are rare in those under age 30.

CAUSES

Diverticula are thought to form over time as the result of weakening in the colon wall where blood vessels exist, much as a weak spot might occur in the wall of an inner tube or tire. Diverticulosis is common in industrialized nations such as the United States and Canada and correspondingly rare in Asia, Africa, and other developing areas. Authorities theorize that a relative lack of dietary fiber in industrialized nations contributes to the development of diverticulosis, which is unseen in countries where whole grains are the largest constituent of diet. The theory is that adding bulk to the stool actually decreases intracolonic pressure, making weak spots and "blowouts" less likely.

SYMPTOMS OF DIVERTICULOSIS

When diverticula occur in the absence of inflammation, the condition is referred to as diverticulosis. Diverticulosis often produces no symptoms. When symptoms do occur, the usual manifestations are episodic, cramping lower abdominal pain, gas, bloating, and irregular bowel movements: symptoms that mimic IBS. Additionally, diverticulosis may occasionally cause rectal bleeding. See your doctor immediately if this occurs.

SYMPTOMS OF DIVERTICULITIS

If a diverticulum ruptures, then intracolonic bacteria are released into the normal sterile abdominal cavity, causing infection and inflammation—referred to as diverticulitis. The symptoms of diverticulitis include fever, abdominal pain, and abdominal tenderness. The pain and tenderness are usually felt in the left lower abdomen, since diverticula are more common in that area of the colon on the left, referred to as the sigmoid colon. Fortunately, diverticulitis is a relatively rare complication of diverticulosis, occurring in fewer than 15 percent of all persons with diverticula.

DIAGNOSIS AND TREATMENT

The presence of diverticula is easily detected by barium-enema X rays or direct observation during endoscopy (sigmoidoscopy or colonoscopy). Treatment for diverticulosis consists of a gradual increase in dietary fiber to decrease intracolonic pressure. Antispasmodics may be used symptomatically to treat the associated cramps. For diverticulitis, antibiotics are prescribed to treat the infection. If oral antibiotics are inadequate, hospitalization, intravenous antibiotics, and occasionally surgery may be required.

TIPS ABOUT FUNCTIONAL DISORDERS AND DISEASES

Remember—a functional disorder is that which has no structural or biochemical explanation for the symptoms. The symptoms are validated by the sufferer, because they are not measured by diagnostic tests. But both functional GI disorders and GI diseases have major impacts on the sufferer's well-being, control of symptoms, and capability of a normal work and social life.

Inflammatory Bowel Disease

Ulcerative colitis and Crohn's disease are chronic inflammatory intestinal conditions of unknown cause. These two disorders are often collectively referred to as inflammatory bowel disease, or IBD. The major difference between the two disorders is that ulcerative colitis is limited to the colon and rectum, whereas Crohn's disease (also referred to as regional enteritis) may affect any segment of the alimentary canal, from the esophagus to the anus. Crohn's disease commonly affects the last portion of the small intestine, referred to as the ileum.

Symptoms of the two disorders are variable, depending on the severity of the disease and which areas are affected. Mild cases are associated with diarrhea and cramping abdominal pain. Bloody diarrhea, fever, and weight loss are seen with more serious cases. Although no clear association exists between IBS and IBD, the symptoms often overlap. Some cases of IBS may represent mild forms of IBD and microscopic evaluation by biopsy of involved areas of the gut may offer the only clue. Furthermore, since both conditions are relatively common, both conditions may occur together in the same individual. Unlike IBS, which does not predispose one to cancer, ulcerative colitis is associated with an increased risk of colon cancer.

The diagnosis of IBD is supported by characteristic X ray findings and is usually confirmed by the pathologist's review of biopsy specimens obtained during endoscopy. Orally and rectally administered corticosteroids are frequently prescribed for treatment as well as various other medications. Surgery may be necessary in severe cases, particularly with ulcerative colitis.

Colon Cancer/Polyps

Some experts contend that in addition to ulcerative colitis, a lack of dietary fiber also predisposes one to the development of colon cancer. Certain types of colon polyps (small, fleshy, mushroom-shaped growths), if left alone, will undergo malignant, cancerous transformation. Colon cancer is very common, with more than 120,000 new cases diagnosed in North America each year. With early detection, the potential for saving lives from this disease is great. The methods of early detection consist of digital rectum exam (in which the physician inserts a gloved index finger into the rectum), testing for occult blood in the stool, and screening sigmoidoscopy or colonoscopy. Some of the presenting symptoms of colon cancer may consist of change in bowel habits, abdominal discomfort, rectal bleeding, weakness secondary to anemia, and weight loss.

The diagnosis is made by X rays or endoscopy of the colon. If premalignant polyps are found, they are usually removed through the colonoscope by a procedure referred to as polypectomy. Follow-up surveillance exams are recommended to detect any recurrences. Colon cancer is usually treated with surgery, sometimes combined with chemotherapy or radiation therapy.

TIPS ABOUT IBS AND COLON CANCER

IBS does not predispose you to colon cancer (or colitis). But it is important for everyone to be aware of colon cancer—the second most frequent cause of death from cancer in North America, after lung cancer. Should your IBS symptoms change and you develop symptoms such as weight loss, bleeding from the rectum, or change in bowel habits or stool caliber, see your doctor immediately! Do not assume it is "simply my IBS."

Appendicitis

While evaluating patients with abdominal pain, I am frequently asked: "Could this be my appendix?" Certainly, this is one of the more common causes of belly pain. Just about everyone knows someone who has had his or her appendix removed. After all, this four-inch dead-end pouch attached to the cecum (the first part of the colon) serves no known useful purpose and frequently becomes infected, causing appendicitis.

Problems of the appendix are not usually chronic and recurring. Rather, acute appendicitis will occur for no particular reason, causing pain that initially is around the umbilicus (belly button) and, as it becomes more intense, will localize to the right lower abdomen. The pain is usually accompanied by fever and a very tender tummy. No special tests are required to make the diagnosis, although an elevated white blood cell count is certainly supportive evidence. When appendicitis is suspected in a relatively sick individual, immediate surgery is usually recommended to remove the appendix before it ruptures.

Hemorrhoids

Hemorrhoids (piles) are one of the more common problems of the digestive tract. Because diarrhea and constipation aggravate the problem, the discomfort of hemorrhoids is especially common in patients with IBS. In addition to causing rectal pain and bleeding, hemorrhoids are a source of embarrassment to many.

I recall one patient who developed a severe case of hemorrhoids while on his honeymoon. It seems he was prone to constipation while traveling, and the constipation, with its resultant straining during bowel movements, resulted in "piles of piles." So much for the horseback riding excursions on that trip!

Frequently patients come in petrified with fear because they have experienced their first bout of rectal bleeding, which turned out to be secondary to hemorrhoids. Although hemorrhoids are a common cause of rectal bleeding, do not assume that they are always the cause. Consult your physician to make certain, as rectal cancer and polyps may also cause bleeding from the rectum. Your doctor may perform an anuscopy or sigmoidoscopy to make this determination.

SYMPTOMS

What, exactly, are hemorrhoids? Simply stated, hemorrhoids are dilated veins around the rectum and anus. When they occur outside the anus they are referred to as external hemorrhoids. The skin overlying external hemorrhoids is very sensitive; therefore, the most common manifestation is pain. A tender lump may be felt when you are bathing.

Internal hemorrhoids occur inside the rectum and do not generally produce pain unless they "pooch out" or prolapse. When internal hemorrhoids prolapse outside the rectum, the anus may close, causing strangulation or thrombosis of the blood vessel. This can be very painful.

Internal hemorrhoids are more likely to bleed, and this may be the only clue to their presence. In addition to pain and bleeding, hemorrhoids may also cause rectal itching when they become irritated, and soiling of the undergarments with mucus or feces, since the swollen veins may prevent complete closure of the anus. Hemorrhoids may be associated with painful anal fissures, which are cracks in the sensitive skin around the anus. Skin tags may form around the anus if the skin overlying the hemorrhoids becomes stretched.

CAUSES

You may be wondering by now what causes hemorrhoids. This is an area of much debate. Conditions that cause increased pressure on the veins in the abdomen, such as pregnancy, are thought to contribute. Varicose

TIPS HOME REMEDIES FOR HEMORRHOIDS

- Avoid constipation or diarrhea. This may be accomplished by increasing dietary fiber. Use of a bulking agent may be helpful in relieving constipation by virtue of its water-retaining properties.

- Avoid straining during bowel movements. When hemorrhoids are present, you may experience a fullness or what is referred to as a sense of incomplete evacuation after a bowel movement. You may push and strain to get this last bit of stool out when, in fact, all of the stool is gone and further straining will only push the hemorrhoids out, causing prolapse.

- Take a sitz bath. Fill the bathtub with just enough very warm water to cover the rectal area. Sit in the tub for a few minutes until the water cools. Do this as often as your schedule permits. Ideally, a sitz bath after each bowel movement would provide optimal cleaning and soothing of the rectal area. If you are plagued with hemorrhoids, consider installing a bidet.

- If you are unable to take a sitz bath or cannot afford to install a bidet, try cleansing with one of the various medicated pads or cotton soaked in witch hazel to help ease discomfort.

veins of the legs are more common with subsequent pregnancies, and hemorrhoids may be likened to varicose veins of the rectum. You can thank your parents for this, since there does seem to be a genetic predisposition to this condition. Straining to pass a large, hard stool, or frequent diarrheal stools, may, as a result of pressure and shearing forces, aggravate the condition. I do not think hemorrhoids are an occupational hazard for truck drivers, but certainly jobs that require prolonged periods of sitting may compound the discomfort.

TREATMENT

Hemorrhoids often respond well to management without medication. See the Table of Home Remedies for treatment options. If these remedies are not sufficient, your doctor may prescribe some hydrocortisone-containing preparations. If all these measures fail, a referral to a surgeon may be indicated for one of the various therapeutic techniques that provide more definitive treatment. Severe pain may develop if a blood clot or thrombosis develops in a hemorrhoid. This occurrence frequently requires surgical intervention.

Proctalgia Fugax

Some people believe that the sudden onset of intense rectal pain—referred to as proctalgia fugax—is in some way related to IBS. There does seem to be a higher incidence of this complaint among IBS sufferers. The pain is usually described as a spasm or a cramp. Although the cause is unknown, symptoms are thought to result from spasm of the muscles around the anus, like a charley horse. A hot sitz bath may relieve the discomfort. Occasionally, medications may be prescribed if symptoms are severe or frequent.

Gallstones

Gallstones are a relatively common cause of abdominal distress. These stones form in a saclike structure called the gallbladder, which is located under the liver. The gallbladder stores the bile manufactured by the liver until it is needed in the small intestine to aid in fat digestion. When called on, the gallbladder contracts to squirt bile into the intestine. If the gallbladder contains stones, the stones may block the flow of bile, resulting in a rather intense pain in the mid-upper or upper right abdomen.

Pain is classically worse after a meal that is high in fat. In less severe cases, nonspecific symptoms such as belching, bloating, and gas may occur: symptoms that commonly occur in IBS patients. The majority of patients with gallstones are asymptomatic, which is to say their gallstones produce no symptoms.

Cholesterol is a major constituent of bile, and most gallstones form because the concentration of cholesterol in the bile is too high. Heredity, advancing age, being a female, and pregnancy are all risk factors for the development of gallstones.

The traditional treatment for symptomatic gallstones has been surgical removal, or cholecystectomy. Recent advances in the treatment of gallstone disease include drugs that slowly dissolve stones, and newer surgical techniques such as laparoscopic laser cholecystectomy. Each of these newer techniques has certain limitations that require individualized recommendations for specific treatment by your physician. If cholecystitis (infection of the gallbladder) develops, then emergency cholecystectomy, using customary techniques, is usually required.

Giardiasis

Infections of the gastrointestinal tract may produce symptoms such as cramps, diarrhea, bloating, and gas. One such infection is due to a common intestinal parasite called *Giardia*. Giardiasis is being recognized more frequently as a cause of acute and chronic illness with higher than average prevalence in the Rocky Mountain region where I practice. The illness may begin suddenly or gradually and may last for days, weeks, or if it becomes chronic, years. Symptoms may occur daily or only intermittently.

For years the presence of *Giardia* in the stool was felt to represent a normal inhabitant of the gut, which did not produce illness. After travel to Russia became more common during the 1970s, where the water source was contaminated, a renewed appreciation of *Giardia* as a cause of gastrointestinal illness occurred. Additionally, it has been observed that *Giardia* may be a source of chronic gastrointestinal complaints lasting years in susceptible individuals and mimicking symptoms of IBS. Common symptoms of chronic *Giardia* include excessive gas, vague abdominal pains, diarrhea and/or constipation, and fatigue. As IBS and *Giardia* are both common these two conditions may occur simultaneously and eradication of *Giardia* may provide lasting improvement. Individuals with underlying IBS who later acquire *Giardia* will become more symptomatic than an individual with normal gut function.

As part of an evaluation of IBS, your doctor may ask you to submit one or several stool specimens so that he or she may look for *Giardia* and other possible causes of gastrointestinal infections. A difficulty arises from the fact that the *Giardia* cyst may be easily missed by standard stool examination. The chance of spotting the cyst is increased by evaluating more than one specimen, but even after three separate specimens are checked, there is approximately a 15-percent chance that diagnosis will be missed in patients with established giardiasis. Fortunately, there is a newer method of stool analysis, which is purported to detect the *Giardia* antigen in most cases with a single stool sample.

As of this writing, there is no definite test to absolutely exclude the possibility of *Giardia*. If giardiasis is suspected, your doctor may elect to prescribe an antibiotic and treat you empirically, without establishing a firm diagnosis. This decision may spare you the trouble of having to play amateur scatologist and study your excrement. It may turn out that as our present knowledge of IBS increases, researchers will discover other intestinal infections that may be the real cause of symptoms in patients previously labeled as having IBS.

CHAPTER 18

Common Tests You May Face

THERE IS NO diagnostic test for IBS—that is, no one test will tell your doctor that you have IBS. However, since IBS can mimic several other more serious conditions, your doctor may ask you to undergo one or more tests. Your doctor will determine which tests are indicated for you based on your symptoms. No one needs to have them all done. All of them, when done properly, should be no more than mildly uncomfortable. This chapter is not exhaustive, but the most commonly performed tests will be reviewed and some of the newer tests that may become more important in the near future will be discussed.

X Rays

UPPER GI SERIES

This test is usually done to be sure you don't have an ulcer in your stomach or duodenum (the first part of your intestine). You will be asked to swallow barium and X rays will be taken of the esophagus, stomach, and duodenum. The entire test usually takes no more than 15 minutes.

BARIUM ENEMA (LOWER GI SERIES)

This test can provide a great deal of information to your doctor. Of course, colon cancer and polyps can be detected, but it also can show diverticulosis, hyperdynamic contractions, a redundant colon, a lax colon, or strictures and other less common conditions. The test is performed by inserting a small tube into the rectum and a balloon is filled with air so it cannot be easily expelled. Barium is then instilled through the tube and

195

the entire colon is filled. When an "air contrast barium enema" is done, air is also instilled for better definition. The test should take only 10 to 15 minutes and you will experience mild cramping and a moderate urge to have a bowel movement.

CAT SCAN

This is a fairly expensive test that takes multiple X rays of the abdomen from different angles, then a computer puts them all together to develop a cross-sectional view of different "slices" of the abdomen. The test is usually performed to look for structural abnormalities of the abdominal organs such as cancer of the liver or pancreas. Usually you will be asked to drink thin barium before the test, and an iodine-based IV contrast will be given. You will be moved through a short tunnel-like structure (about three feet long). The test takes between 10 and 30 minutes and is painless.

MRI

Like a CAT scan, magnetic resonance imaging (MRI) is usually performed to look for structural abnormalities of the abdominal organs. The detail of images provided by MRI is usually superior to the CAT scan. The test takes between 10 to 15 minutes. Since magnets are used for the test, it cannot be performed in patients who have artificial metal implants, such as a metal hip prosthesis.

ULTRASOUND

This test is done by passing ultrasound waves through your abdomen. Usually, the gallbladder, liver, pancreas, and kidney are examined. No radiation is involved and the test should take no more than 10 to 20 minutes. It is painless, but some pressure is felt because the ultrasound probe must be firmly pressed against the abdomen.

COLON TRANSIT TEST

This simple test is utilized to evaluate the movement of intestinal contents through the colon in constipated patients. It involves ingestion of several small rings that are easily seen on plain X rays, which are taken a few days after the rings are ingested. Normal colon transit is suggested if none of the rings are present. If the rings are dispersed diffusely throughout the colon, decreased colonic motility is suggested. If all the rings have accumulated near the rectum, a possible mechanical obstruction of the lower bowel may be present.

Nuclear Medicine

GASTRIC EMPTYING STUDY

More and more we are coming to realize that many of the symptoms of IBS are due to motility disturbances (that is, contraction and relaxation of the gut). Nausea, vomiting, abdominal fullness, and ulcer pain in the absence of any ulcer can all be caused by stomach and upper small intestine dysmotility (abnormal motility).

For this test, you will be asked to eat a small amount of food that has a minute amount of radioactive material attached to it. By using extremely sensitive scanners, the meal can be seen in the stomach and the time it takes for the stomach to empty can be determined. If the test shows slow emptying, your doctor can give you medicines that can normalize it. The test is painless and takes 60 to 90 minutes to perform. The radioactivity you receive is about the same dose as for a routine chest X ray.

Endoscopy

UPPER ENDOSCOPY

This is also called an EGD for esophagogastroduodenoscopy. In order to do the test, you must fast overnight. An IV will be inserted into a vein so that sedative medication can be given. After you are asleep, a thin tube that can send a picture to a television screen will be placed into your mouth and then into the esophagus. The doctor doing the test will be able to see your esophagus, stomach, and upper small intestine. Biopsies can be done if necessary (you have no pain nerves here so it won't hurt and you shouldn't be sore afterward).

This is by far the best test to look for ulcers, esophagitis, and gastritis, but it is also expensive and relatively invasive so your doctor will order it only in selected cases. The sedation time is usually 5 to 10 minutes, the endoscopy takes 5 to 15 minutes and the recovery (waking-up time) is 20 to 30 minutes.

THE COLON

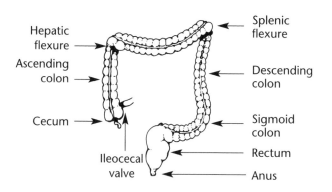

Hepatic flexure

Ascending colon

Cecum

Ileocecal valve

Splenic flexure

Descending colon

Sigmoid colon

Rectum

Anus

Reproduced with permission from the
International Foundation for Functional Gastrointestinal Disorders.

COLONOSCOPY

This is the best test to look for cancer and polyps, and should discover over 95 percent of them. If a polyp is found, it can be removed at the same time; this is a painless procedure since you have no pain nerves in the lining of your colon. As with the upper endoscopy, an IV is placed so that sedation can be given. The test generally takes 30 to 60 minutes and the waking-up time is 20 to 30 minutes. Given proper sedation, the test should not be uncomfortable. The colon must be very clean to do the test and therefore laxatives must be given beforehand to purge completely.

FLEXIBLE SIGMOIDOSCOPY

This test is like a colonoscopy, but the tube that is inserted is much shorter, and only enemas are needed to prepare the colon. It is often done in your physician's office and doesn't require an IV or sedation. The test can quickly tell your doctor if you have inflammation of your colon or if bleeding is coming from the lower part of the colon. Biopsies can be done (again, painlessly).

The test should take only 5 to 10 minutes in experienced hands, and generally you will only feel some gas and moderate cramping. Some patients with IBS are more sensitive to bowel distention and stretching and can be momentarily more uncomfortable.

Blood Tests

CBC (CELL BLOOD COUNT)

This is a blood count. It tells your doctor if you're anemic, if your white cell count is high (possibly indicating an infection), and other aspects of your blood. If you are anemic, other tests may need to be done.

CHEMISTRY PANEL

This test provides a wealth of information to your doctor. It shows how much salt and potassium (which can be lost with diarrhea) are present, how the liver is functioning, and even gives a very general picture of your nutrition. Thyroid hormone levels may indicate an underactive thyroid (which may underlie constipation) or an overactive thyroid (manifesting as frequent bowel movements or diarrhea).

ANTIGLIADEN ANTIBODIES

Celiac sprue is a partially understood disease that has a very insidious onset. It is caused by a sensitivity (not an allergy) to gluten, a component of certain grains, such as wheat, barley, and oats. In this disease, the cells in the small intestine that are responsible for absorbing food lose their ability to absorb nutrients. This results in the slow onset of malabsorption and, ultimately, malnutrition. Early symptoms can be bloating, increasingly audible bowel sounds, and loose stools. Since these may be the same symptoms that many patients with IBS experience, the diagnosis could be falsely attributed to IBS.

Currently, the only definitive way to make the diagnosis is by biopsying the small intestine during the upper endoscopy test (EGD). Other antibody blood tests have recently been developed, and may be more valuable in making a diagnosis of gluten sensitivity than antigliaden antibodies.

H. PYLORI ANTIBODIES

In the past few years, we have come to understand that most ulcers are actually caused or perpetuated by a bacterium *(Helicobacter pylori)* that lives in the stomach. Your body develops antibodies to *H. pylori* if you are infected, which can be discovered by a blood test.

Research into this area is rapidly changing our understanding of the diseases and symptoms caused by this bacterium. At present, we know that it can cause gastritis (irritation of the stomach lining without ulceration) and ulceration of the stomach or intestine. However, it can also be present when there are no ulcers or gastritis, in patients who have ulcer-like symptoms (nonulcer dyspepsia).

STOOL TESTS

Giardia is a parasite that lives in the small bowel. As discussed in the previous chapter, it can cause severe diarrhea when the infection is acute. Chronically it can cause more subtle symptoms, such as intermittent bloating, flatulence, and loose stools. Testing of stool samples for antigens (parts of the organism) has proven useful; it can even pick up cases of infection when the microscopic examination of the stool is negative. Presently, most doctors and labs make the diagnosis of *Giardia* by having specially trained technicians look at stool specimens for eggs or parasites. Human error or low concentrations of parasite can lead to "false-negatives," which means a test is reported as negative when the patient really has the disease. Other parasitic infections of the intestinal tract may be discovered by microscopic analysis of stool specimens.

Diagnostic Questionnaires

THE HALLMARK OF IBS is abdominal pain or discomfort. This pain or discomfort is associated with an altered pattern of bowel movement—usually a tendency towards diarrhea, constipation, or a pattern characterized by diarrhea alternating with constipation.

The following are two questionnaires: the first is a checklist that may be helpful for you to determine whether or not you may have IBS. *Remember, this information is not a substitute for the advice and guidance of a qualified health-care practitioner.* The second questionnaire is a much more detailed checklist of questions that your primary care physician will most likely ask.

Do You Have IBS? A Checklist for You

Symptoms that suggest IBS (check those that apply to you):

❑ Abdominal pain or discomfort
❑ Relief of the abdominal pain or discomfort with the passage of stool
❑ Onset of abdominal pain or discomfort associated with a change in stool frequency
❑ Onset of abdominal pain or discomfort associated with a change in form (appearance) of stool
❑ Passage of mucus during a bowel movement
❑ A feeling of abdominal fullness, swelling, or bloating

❑ A feeling the rectum is not empty after a bowel movement
❑ A sense of urgency associated with a bowel movement
❑ Less than three bowel movements a week
❑ More than three bowel movements a day
❑ A stool that is hard and difficult to pass
❑ Loose, unformed, or watery bowel movements

Symptoms that suggest a condition other than IBS (check those that apply to you):

❑ Onset of symptoms later in life (after age 45)
❑ Weight loss
❑ Fever
❑ Passage of blood in the stool
❑ Awakening at night as the result of symptoms
❑ Family history of colon cancer, colon polyps, inflammatory bowel disorders

IBS Questionnaire for Consultation with Your Physician

Following is a detailed questionnaire that I have utilized over the years to evaluate patients referred to me for possible IBS. Completion of the section may facilitate a discussion of your symptoms with your physician. It also may help you to think about and characterize your specific complaints. Questions marked with an asterisk refer to "Helpful Hints" included after this section.

1. How long have you had abdominal pain? _____
2. Do you have more than one pain? Yes ❑   No ❑   If so, how many different pains do you have?_____
3. Where is the worst pain? Left lower abdomen ❑   Left upper abdomen ❑   Right lower abdomen ❑   Right upper abdomen ❑
4. How often does the pain occur, and how long does it generally last?
   _____
5. Does the pain ever awaken you from sleep?* Yes ❑   No ❑
6. Do you ever awaken from sleep because of diarrhea?* Yes ❑   No ❑

7. Is the pain ever so severe that it is unbearable and interferes with your normal daily activities? Yes ❑ No ❑

8. On a scale of 1 (no pain) to 10 (unbearable pain), how would you rate your pain at its worst? _____

9. How would you describe the pain? Cramping ❑ Aching ❑ Burning ❑ Knifelike ❑ Other: _____

10. Have you found anything you can do or take to alleviate the pain?
_____

11. Does eating or drinking make the pain worse? Yes ❑ No ❑

12. Have you identified certain foods that seem to trigger pain or diarrhea? If so, please list those foods: _____
_____

13. Describe your typical pattern of bowel movements and the consistency of feces (e.g., one bowel movement, every three days, which is hard and difficult to pass; or two or three loose, watery bowel movements a day): _____
_____

14. How did your digestive symptoms develop? Suddenly ❑ Gradually ❑
If sudden, describe the circumstances and symptoms at the time of initial onset: _____
_____

15. Has this pattern remained constant, or has it changed in recent months?* _____
_____

16. Is the pain usually relieved after a bowel movement? Yes ❑ No ❑

17. Do you have a change in the frequency or form (appearance) of bowel movement at the onset of pain? Yes ❑ No ❑ If yes, check the following that applies at the onset of pain: More loose ❑ More frequent ❑ Less frequent ❑ More hard ❑ Difficult to pass ❑

18. Do you have any of the following associated symptoms?*
Bloating ❑ Belching ❑ Gas ❑ Nausea ❑ Vomiting ❑

19. Have you passed mucus in your stool? Yes ❑   No ❑

20. Have you lost weight in recent months?* If so, how much, over what period of time, and to what do you attribute the weight loss?

_____

_____

21. Have you passed blood in your stool, or had any black, tarry bowel movements?* Yes ❑   No ❑

22. Have you ever had fever associated with your symptoms?* Yes ❑ No ❑

23. Have you previously been evaluated for these complaints? If so, what tests were performed, and what were the results? _____

_____

_____

24. Comment on the effectiveness or side effects of any previously pre-scribed medications that you have taken for your complaints:

_____

_____

_____

25. Have you ever been told you have IBS, or spastic colon? Yes ❑ No ❑

26. Do you often feel nervous or anxious?* Yes ❑   No ❑

27. Does stress make your IBS symptoms worse?* Yes ❑   No ❑

28. Do you often feel sad or depressed?* Yes ❑   No ❑

29. Are you currently receiving mental health care?* Yes ❑   No ❑

30. Have you ever received mental health care?* Yes ❑   No ❑

31. Are you currently taking psychiatric medications?* Yes ❑   No ❑

32. Have you ever felt suicidal or self-destructive?* Yes ❑   No ❑

33. Do you have frequent dreams or recurrent nightmares?* Yes ❑ No ❑

34. Have you ever had a black-out or lost time?* Yes ❑   No ❑

35. Have you ever been the victim of physical or sexual abuse?* Yes ❑ No ❑

36. Do you ever become fearful or anxious when out in public?* Yes ❑ No ❑

37. Have you ever had headaches caused from various foods?* Yes ❑ No ❑ If yes, please list those foods: _____

_____

_____

38. Do you have any other medical problems you would consider un-controlled at this time? Yes ❑ No ❑ If yes, please list those prob-lems: _____

_____

_____

39. Have you had your gallbladder removed?* Yes ❑ No ❑

40. Have you ever had, or been treated for, *Giardia*? Yes ❑ No ❑

41. Do you have frequent pains in the neck, shoulders and back?* Yes ❑ No ❑

42. Describe your energy level:* Poor ❑ Fair ❑ Good ❑ Excellent ❑

43. Do you have cravings for certain foods?* Yes ❑ No ❑ If yes, please list those foods: _____

_____

_____

44. Do you regularly consume any of the following? Check those that apply: Fruit juices ❑ Sodas ❑ Diet sodas ❑ Dietetic foods ❑ Foods with artificial sweeteners ❑ Gum or mints ❑ Carbonated beverages ❑ Foods with MSG or "flavor enhancers" ❑

For Female Patients Only

45. Are you pregnant, or do you think you might be? Yes ❑ No ❑

46. Do your digestive symptoms worsen prior to the onset of your men-strual period? Yes ❑ No ❑

47. Do you have pain with intercourse? Yes ❑ No ❑

Helpful Hints about the IBS Questionnaire

*5, 6. Symptoms of IBS do not occur at night.

*15. IBS symptoms usually remain constant; a change in the pattern re-quires consultation with your physician to exclude a new disorder.

*18. If you have belching, bloating, or gas, refer to Chapter 15.

*20–22. Weight loss, blood in bowel movements, and fever are "red flags" that suggest another disorder requiring evaluation by your physician.

*26–36. These questions are designed to elicit symptoms of coexisting psychological problems that need to be addressed as part of a total IBS treatment plan. Refer to Chapter 11.

*37. MSG-sensitive people may have coexisting headaches (particularly migraine). Avoidance of MSG often helps to reduce headaches and IBS symptoms as well. Refer to Chapters 4 and 5.

*39. Patients with diarrhea-predominant IBS-like symptoms who have had their gallbladder removed may respond well to medications that bind excessive bile acids. Refer to Chapter 14.

*41, 42. Positive responses to these questions suggest possible coexisting FMS. Refer to Chapter 16.

*43. Often foods that we crave or consume on a regular basis may be dietary triggers that should be avoided on a trial basis.

Common Questions and Answers About IBS

QUESTION: What causes IBS?

ANSWER: Although the exact cause of IBS is not known, there seems to exist an underlying abnormality that results in the disruption of normal rhythmic contractions of the intestinal tract. Abdominal pain and altered bowel function (variations of diarrhea or constipation) are the symptoms experienced when intestinal contractions are disrupted. Emotional stress and certain foods lead the list of factors that may trigger symptoms. Genetic predisposition as well as recurrent abdominal pains during childhood may predispose one to the development of this disorder.

QUESTION: Can stress alone cause IBS?

ANSWER: Stress can be the primary cause of symptoms in some IBS sufferers and physicians may suggest they try stress management and relaxation techniques or see a therapist for help. Chronic stress is responsible for a number of symptoms such as tension headaches, chest discomfort, fatigue, muscle aches, and susceptibility to infection. This kind of stress may also predispose individuals to functional disorders such as IBS.

QUESTION: How is the diagnosis of IBS made?

ANSWER: Unfortunately, there is no conclusive test to firmly establish a diagnosis of IBS. The diagnosis is suggested by a specific set of symptoms or criteria such as the Rome II criteria, which, simply stated, includes abdominal pain associated with altered bowel movements. Physical examination, blood tests, stool specimens, X rays, and endoscopy may be used to exclude other diseases or disorders that produce symptoms similar to IBS.

QUESTION: How is IBS treated?

ANSWER: Treatment begins with patient education. It is important to develop an understanding of what is and what is not known about IBS and the underlying intestinal rhythmic disorder. Appropriate lifestyle changes such as dietary changes, stress reduction, and exercise should be made. Appropriate remedies or medications may be prescribed to treat certain aspects of the disorder. Ideally, a cooperative team approach will be developed with your physician to help you gain control over your IBS symptoms.

QUESTION: Is there a cure for IBS?

ANSWER: There is as yet no cure for IBS in the same sense that a course of antibiotics may cure an infection. IBS will often cause periodic symptoms, with symptom-free intervals lasting days, months, or years. However, you can learn to gain control over your symptoms, thereby increasing the symptom-free intervals. To the extent that you are able to remain symptom free by following and refining the suggestions outlined in this book, you may actually experience a "cure."

QUESTION: What is the difference between colitis and IBS?

ANSWER: The term "colitis" implies inflammation of the colon. IBS is not associated with colon inflammation and should not be confused with inflammatory bowel disease (IBD). IBD sufferers will often have bloody diarrhea, fever, and weight loss—symptoms associated with colon inflammation.

QUESTION: Will IBS predispose me to more serious disorders?
ANSWER: No, having IBS will not make you more likely to develop such conditions as inflammatory bowel disease, colon cancer, or colon polyps. And IBS will not require surgery. At the same time, managing your IBS well will not protect you from developing other bowel conditions, and if you see any change in your usual pattern of symptoms, you should consult your physician.

QUESTION: Will my children be prone to IBS if I have it?
ANSWER: It does appear from scientific evidence that a parental history of functional GI disorders may predispose children to having similar health problems. However, learned attitudes and behavior may be just as influential as genetics. What is most important for parents to be aware of is how they cope with IBS. If you try to maintain a "normal" lifestyle by gaining control of your IBS symptoms, you will be an excellent model for your child, who may possibly face this challenge in the future.

QUESTION: What are the warning signs that something other than IBS is going on?
ANSWER: A partial list of worrisome symptoms includes fever, weight loss, anemia, painful or difficult swallowing, persistent vomiting, a sense of feeling full sooner than usual during meals, new or different pains, symptoms of pain and abnormal bowel function occurring at night, persistent diarrhea, worsening constipation, rectal bleeding, or blood in the stool. If any of these symptoms occur, contact your doctor. When your doctor undertakes a detailed clinical history and physical exam to make a diagnosis, he or she will look for other "red flags," such as if your symptoms began at the age of 50 years or older (IBS usually begins earlier in life), and if you have a family history of digestive tract cancer, inflammatory bowel disease, or celiac disease.

QUESTION: Are there tests for lactose intolerance?
ANSWER: Yes, the hydrogen breath test is a simple, effective test, usually conducted at the GI lab of a hospital, to determine an inability to com-

pletely digest the sugar lactose found in dairy products. The test, which takes two to three hours, involves ingestion of lactose and the periodic analysis of expired air. If lactose is not completely digested and absorbed in the intestinal tract, it will eventually end up in the colon, where it will be fermented by colonic bacteria. During this process, above-normal amounts of hydrogen gas are produced, some of which is absorbed into the bloodstream and later expired through the lungs.

QUESTION: Should I take calcium supplements if I have a lactose intolerance?

ANSWER: If you have a lactose intolerance and for this reason avoid dairy products, you should take calcium supplements. You should take between 1000 and 1500 milligrams of calcium daily. Taking calcium supplements with vitamin D or a multiple vitamin that contains vitamin D will improve absorption. Alternatively, persons with lactose intolerance may tolerate dairy products by taking lactase enzyme supplements when they are eating dairy products.

QUESTION: Do spicy foods make IBS symptoms worse?

ANSWER: Spicy foods sometimes make IBS symptoms worse but not always. For example, many patients have told me they cannot tolerate Mexican food because it is "too spicy." Further investigation has revealed it was the high fat content of the average Mexican meal (fried chips, cheese, refried beans, sour cream, guacamole) rather than the hot, spicy salsa that triggered the symptoms. These patients can enjoy modified Mexican, Cajun, and similar entrees that have reduced fat but retain their distinctive spices.

QUESTION: Are herbs useful for treating IBS symptoms?

ANSWER: Herbal therapy can be effective for relief of IBS symptoms. At least one study looked at Chinese herbs and found that a standardized preparation and an individualized preparation were more effective than placebo. Remember that herbs, like medications, may have side effects and the potential for interaction with medications.

QUESTION: Is there a relationship between IBS and sexual dysfunction?
ANSWER: One study suggests that women with IBS are more likely to complain of uncomfortable intercourse than women with peptic ulcer disease. The explanation for this finding might be that abdominal cramps, gas, and bloating make intercourse less pleasurable and thus lessen sexual gratification. Many women have reported enhanced sexuality with mastery and control of their IBS symptoms.

QUESTION: How can therapy help with IBS?
ANSWER: There are a variety of therapies that bring relief of IBS symptoms, and most deal with underlying factors that contribute to IBS. Both biofeedback and cognitive behavioral therapy reveal how cognitive-behavioral patterns produce physiological changes. If you have problems of anxiety or depression, for example, the body habitually responds to circumstances with alarm, fear, or overload—the same effects of chronic stress. A range of medications is available to treat all forms of anxiety, but to alleviate IBS symptoms for the long-term, it is most effective to uncover the underlying causes of your distress.

Lactose-Free Diet

Lactose intolerance or sensitivity, like many other food intolerances and sensitivities, is quantitative as well as qualitative. Most lactose-intolerant individuals become symptomatic (experiencing gas, cramps, bloating, and diarrhea) after ingesting 12 grams of lactose. This is the approximate content of an eight-ounce glass of milk. Some people, particularly those with IBS and lactose intolerance, may become symptomatic after as little as three grams of lactose. Lactose may be better tolerated when taken with other foods. Small amounts of butter and cheese may be tolerated, depending on the individual.

Read labels carefully! Avoid any product that contains milk, milk products, milk solids, whey, casein, curd, lactose, or galactose. Small amounts of these substances may be tolerated; however, the quantity of lactose may not be stated on the label.

Lactase enzyme supplements may be used to treat milk to decrease the lactose content or may be taken with milk or lactose-containing products. Lactase-treated milk is sweeter than regular milk.

Lactose-intolerant individuals who avoid all dairy products should take calcium supplements. Usually 1000 to 1500 milligrams of elemental calcium should be taken daily.

Following is a comprehensive listing of common foods to avoid and those that are allowed, depending on the severity of your lactose intolerance.

LACTOSE-FREE DIET

Type of Food	Foods Allowed	Foods to Avoid
Milk or milk products	Nondairy products that do not contain lactose. Soybean milk may be used as a substitute.	All milk or milk products as listed on the previous page. For example: yogurt, cheese, ice cream, sherbet.
Eggs	All.	None.
Vegetables	All (organic vegetables are preferable where available).	Vegetables prepared with foods to avoid such as cream, margarine, butter.
Meat, fish, poultry	All types of meat, fish, and poultry that are not creamed or breaded.	Creamed or breaded meat, fish, or poultry. Luncheon meats, sausage, and any processed meat that contains milk products.
Bread, grains, and cereals	All products that do not contain milk or milk products.	All products containing milk or milk products.
Fats	All types of fats that do not contain milk or milk products.	Butter, margarine, sour cream, or any product that contains milk or milk products.
Soups	Those broth-based soups that do not contain milk or milk products.	Cream soups or any soups that contain milk or milk products.
Fruits and fruit juices	All fresh, frozen, or canned products without lactose (organic fruit preferable where available).	Any product prepared with lactose.
Desserts	Angel food cake, Jell-O, sorbets, or any product made without milk products.	Most commercial desserts and any product made with milk or milk products.
Miscellaneous	Nuts, peanut butter, pure sugar, and honey.	All gravies, sauces, candies, liqueurs, or commercial mixers made with milk or milk products, molasses.

How to Stop Smoking

CIGARETTE SMOKING is the greatest single cause of chronic illness, disability, and death in North America. If you have IBS and smoke, you can quit. Stopping smoking may be the most difficult lifestyle change you need to make to improve your IBS symptoms and overall health. For this reason, I have included this appendix.

Cigarette smoking threatens a smoker's survival, decreases energy levels, increases risk of heart disease, lung disease, and cancer, and decreases his or her ability to fight infection. Secondhand smoke also threatens a smoker's spouse, children, coworkers, and friends.

Now that the U.S. surgeon general has declared nicotine an "addictive" drug, you can count on an increased number of quick cures and products for those seeking to quit. In fact, there are numerous programs and products with little proven success, designed primarily to separate you from your money. The unfortunate fact is that there is no quick or easy route to permanent independence from tobacco. To successfully quit smoking, you must be aware of two aspects of your habits: your associative habits and your dependence on nicotine.

Associative habits are those you have developed over the years. Smoking may be particularly satisfying with coffee, after a meal, first thing in the morning, with a drink in the evening, and so on. Many smokers overcome this habit by waiting for a short period after the associative activity before smoking a cigarette. For example, have the cup of coffee, wait half an hour, then have the cigarette. If you're one of those who reach for that pack as soon as they rise, then get up, wait a half hour, then have your first cigarette. The secret is to break up these associative habits, whatever they are. Do one activity, then the other.

To overcome a dependence on nicotine, seek brands with increasingly lower nicotine content. Most brands that are lower in tars and nicotine list their comparative contents, either on the package or in their advertisements. This should be a well-thought-out process so that you know what brand you will be going to next. Do not go to the lowest nicotine all at once; to be successful, you need a gradual withdrawal of your dependence.

Some people prefer to quit cold turkey. This technique is often effective but may increase the intensity of nicotine withdrawal symptoms—namely, irritability and anxiety. An advantage to this approach, however, is that the entire process is shortened. I encourage my patients who have had to quit for various reasons, such as an illness requiring hospitalization, to not resume the habit, since they have already gone through the withdrawal period.

Some authorities insist it is best to set a target date for quitting, say, six to eight weeks from the time you decide to quit. Then tell everyone about that date. ("On September 25, I will stop smoking.") Others find setting a date an additional stress. Remember, you are seeking to achieve something permanently beneficial to your health. If you have been smoking for several years, the few weeks or months you devote to a concerted effort to quit are well worth the struggle. You emerge a winner.

Seek the advice of your physician. New practices or methods may be available that are well worth exploring. For example, Wellbutrin (Zyban) is a medication previously used to treat depression that has been shown to be successful in helping some smokers stop. Additionally, there are a multitude of nicotine substitutes that may be used to decrease the physical cravings while you try to break the habit.

There are a number of professionally run clinics and groups sponsored by medical centers and hospitals. Many of my patients have found the Hooked But Not Helpless program, which addresses the psychological factors associated with nocotine addiction, worthwhile (www.stop smoking.com). Perhaps there are several in your area. You may want to join one for support and suggestions. The American Cancer Society has a wealth of information and some sound policies and practices for those who want to quit smoking. Contact and support your local branch.

After you have made up your mind to quit, try to maintain as nearly normal a schedule as possible and avoid stressful situations whenever possible while attempting to quit.

What if you fail? Many smokers have failed in their first attempts to quit. Do not be discouraged. Studies indicate that with repeated attempts, the probability of success actually increases.

Don't worry about gaining weight. Perhaps you'll gain 10 to 15 pounds, mainly because food tastes better and you enjoy the oral gratification achieved through eating rather than smoking. But weight is much easier to deal with than smoking, and as a nonsmoker, you will learn to relish more healthful snacks and discover increased energy through exercise.

Once you feel you have become independent of nicotine and cigarettes, or you reach your target date, try to take a weekend away from your normal environment. Leave your partially consumed pack or your partial carton at home and try to enjoy yourself. If you live in the city, go to the country; if your home is in the mountains, visit the city. It is only normal to have a twinge of longing for that cigarette, but try not to dwell on that need. Keep busy; try some different foods, or a new activity. It may also be beneficial to avoid places where smoking is prevalent for a few weeks, until you have had a chance to establish your new lifestyle.

Once you have truly kicked your dependence, celebrate it each year. Make the anniversary of the day you finally quit for good "Mike's Day" or "Sally's Day." This is your day. Take it off from work. Do exactly what you want to do. Spend your time with those you want to see; eat the foods you enjoy. Celebrate. You've earned it.

Resources

Stress and IBS
• a tape cassette with information on IBS and help to relax
www.ibsinformation.com

International Foundation for Functional Gastrointestinal Disorders (IFFGD)
PO Box 170864
Milwaukee, WI 53217
www.iffgd.org, iffgd@iffgd.org
1-888-964-2001

Food and Drug Administration
Center for Drug Evaluation and Research
www.fda.gov/cder/drug/infopage

National Institutes of Health
www.nih.gov

National Institute of Mental Health
6001 Executive Blvd.
Room 8184 MSC 9663
Bethesda, MD 20892-9663
www.nimh.nih.gov
1-800-647-2642
• for information on panic disorder, phobias, depression, etc.

National Center for Complementary and Alternative Medicine
NCCAM Clearinghouse
PO Box 8218
Silver Spring, MD 20907-8218
nccam.nih.gov
1-888-644-6226

Chronic Fatigue and Immune
Dysfunction Syndrome (CFIDS)
Association of America
PO Box 220398
Charlotte, NC 28222-0398
www.cfids.org
1-800-442-3437

National Headache Foundation
428 West St. James Place
Chicago, IL 60614
www.headaches.org
1-800-843-2256

Obsessive-Compulsive
Foundation
www.ocdresource.com
1-800-NEWS-4-OCD

Anxiety Disorders Association
of America
11900 Parklawn Dr., #100
Rockville, MD 20852-2624
www.adaa.org
301-231-9350

BEANO
AkPharma Inc.
www.akpharma.com
1-800-GET-BEANO

Lactaid
• a lactase enzyme for lactose
intolerance
AkPharma Inc.
www.akpharma.com
1-800-LACTAID

KYOLIC BESURE
• for anti-flatulence and digestive
support products
Blessed Nutrition Inc.
www.blessednutrition.com
1-800-688-3933

Flatulence Filter
• an air filter inside a chair
cushion
Ultra Tech Products Inc.
www.flatulencefilter.com
1-800-316-8668

American Holistic Medical
Association
6728 Old McLean Village Drive
McLean, VA 22101-3906
703-556-9728

American Botanical Council
PO Box 201660
Austin, TX 78720
512-331-8868

Information and links to CAM research:
www.1healthyuniverse.com
• Annual updates on evidence-based research, with over 3500 references to all CAM disciplines

The Scientific Basis for Holistic Medicine: Annotated Abstracts
by Bob Anderson, M.D.
Clinical Pathways, Inc.
1180 Claremont St.
Denver, CO 80220

Great Smokies Diagnostic Laboratory
63 Zillicoa St.
Asheville, NC 28801-1074
1-800-522-4762

By courtesy of Paul Donovan, Ph.D., for most of this information

Glossary

Acetylcholine—an important neurotransmitter in the body that is responsible for transmission of nerve impulses throughout the parasympathetic branch of the autonomic nervous system.

Aerobic exercise—any prolonged, rhythmical exercise that uses major muscle groups. Aerobic exercises require oxygen and increase heart rate and respiratory rate.

Aerophagia—habitual swallowing of air.

Alimentary canal—all of the organs making up the route taken by food as it passes through the body from the mouth to the anus.

Allergy—an abnormal and individual sensitivity to substances that are usually harmless. Traditionally, allergy occurs when the body's preformed antibodies make contact with the offending substance (the allergen), resulting in the allergic reaction.

Amphetamine—usually a white, crystalline powder that stimulates the nervous system.

Amylase—the enzyme responsible for the breakdown of complex carbohydrates into simpler compounds.

Anemia—a deficiency in the quality or quantity of red blood cells.

Antacid—medication used to neutralize stomach acid.

Antispasmodic—medication used to treat intestinal spasms.

Appendectomy—surgical removal of the appendix.

Appendicitis—inflammation or infection of the appendix. The appendix is a 4-inch, dead-end pouch attached to the cecum (the first part of the colon).

Arteriosclerosis—thickening and loss of elasticity of the wall of the arteries, frequently referred to as "hardening of the arteries."

Autonomic nervous system—that branch of the nervous system that works without conscious control. The autonomic nervous system has two subdivisions: the sympathetic system and the parasympathetic system.

Barium—a chalky liquid that is either swallowed or inserted into the rectum during X ray procedures to outline or contrast the lining of the intestinal tract.

Barium enema (lower GI)—an X ray examination of the colon. During this exam, barium (a chalky liquid) is inserted into the rectum to contrast and outline the colon.

Beta blocker—the class of medications that block the beta receptors in the body. The beta receptors are activated by the neurotransmitter adrenalin.

Bile—a clear yellow or orange fluid produced by the liver that is concentrated and stored in the gallbladder until needed for digestion. The bile salts help to break up large molecules of fat into smaller molecules that may be absorbed by the body.

Biofeedback—the use of electronic equipment to display and monitor bodily functions for the purpose of modifying them and reducing symptoms of a variety of disorders, including functional GI disorders.

Biopsychosocial model—a re-emerging approach to medicine and research that integrates the mind, body, and environment into the cause and effect of health and illness.

Bolus—the soft mass of chewed food that enters the esophagus with each swallow.

Brain-gut connection—the connection between the central and enteric nervous systems in the functioning of the gastrointestinal tract.

Bulking agent—an agent that gives bulk to the stool.

Caffeine—a white powder found naturally in coffee and tea that acts as a stimulant to the central nervous system and as a mild diuretic.

Calisthenics—exercises for developing bodily strength and gracefulness.

Casein—a protein found in milk and other dairy products.

Cholycystectomy—surgical removal of the gallbladder.

Cholecystogram—an X ray of the gallbladder taken after the ingestion of tablets that provide contrast of the gallbladder.

Cholecystokinin—a hormone secreted in the small intestine that stimulates contraction of the gallbladder and the colon.

Chyme—a material produced by the action of gastric secretions on ingested food, which is then discharged from the stomach into the first part of the small intestine, called the duodenum.

Clinical history—a patient/physician interview during which detailed information regarding symptoms and past medical problems is obtained.

Cognitive behavioral therapy—a therapeutic method to identify and modify automatic patterns of thinking, feeling, and reacting.

Colic—pertaining to the colon. "Colic" usually refers to attacks of abdominal pain that are thought to result from spasms of the intestines. Colic occurs most frequently in infants.

Colon—the part of the large intestine extending from the small intestine to the rectum.

Colonoscopy—endoscopic (see Endoscopy) or direct visualization of the entire colon utilizing a fiber optic scope, referred to as a colonoscope.

Colon polyp—a small, fleshy, mushroom-shaped growth occurring in the colon. Certain types of colon polyps are believed to undergo cancerous transformation if not removed.

Complex carbohydrate—a large molecule consisting of simple carbohydrates or simple sugars linked together. Complex carbohydrates are found in grains, fruits, vegetables, and "starchy" foods (such as bread, rice, pasta), among other foods.

Complementary alternative medicine—a practice of health care in which the mind, body, and environment are treated as interconnected. Preventive health care is a common feature of CAM therapies, which include acupuncture, chiropractic, traditional Chinese medicine, Ayurveda, aromatherapy, herbal therapy, homeopathy, and biofeedback.

Crohn's disease—a form of inflammatory bowel disease also referred to as regional enteritis, which involves inflammation of the intestinal tract (frequently the last portion of the small intestine, known as the ileum).

Cruciferous vegetables—a family of plants including broccoli, cabbage, cauliflower, and brussels sprouts that cause intestinal gas due to the presence of lactose, fructose, sorbitol, and raffinose in these vegetables.

Defecation—the elimination of wastes and undigested food as feces from the anus.

Diagnosis—the art or method of identifying or recognizing disease.

Digestion—the process whereby food is broken down into smaller units suitable for absorption into the blood and utilization by the body's individual cells.

Diverticulitis—inflammation of diverticula. Symptoms of diverticulitis may include abdominal pain, usually in the left lower abdomen, and fever.

Diverticulosis—the presence of diverticula.

Diverticulum—a small blind pouch that forms in the wall of the colon.

Duodenum—the first portion of the small intestine, which is usually approximately 10 inches long.

Elimination diet—a diet used for diagnosing food allergies or sensitivities, based on omission of foods that might cause symptoms.

Emulsifier—a substance used to break up and mix two liquids that under ordinary circumstances will not mix—such as oil and water. Detergents act as emulsifiers by breaking up grease, which may then mix with water. Bile acids, produced by the liver, are also emulsifiers, since they aid in digestion by breaking up fats in the intestinal tract, making them suitable for absorption into the bloodstream.

Endorphin—a naturally occurring protein produced in the brain that has a pain-relieving "morphinelike" effect. Among other things, endorphins are thought to mediate the so-called runner's high.

Endoscopy—the visual examination of the interior structures of the body through a lighted fiber optic instrument referred to as an endoscope.

Enteric nervous system—or "gut brain," a part of the autonomic nervous system that controls and coordinates the digestive process by regulating such things as smooth muscle contraction, blood flow to the digestive organs, and movement of fluids and electrolytes in the intestines.

Eructation (belching)—the oral ejection of air from the stomach.

Esophageal spasm—a cramplike pain, usually in the center of the chest, produced by spasms of the esophagus.

Esophagogastroduodenoscopy (EGD)—direct observation of the esophagus, stomach, and duodenum through a lighted fiber optic instrument referred to as an endoscope.

Esophagus—that portion of the alimentary canal that extends from the back of the throat to the stomach. In an average adult, it usually measures 10 to 12 inches long.

Exercise stress test—a continuous monitoring of the heart's electrical activity during exercise to ascertain exercise tolerance and the presence of underlying heart abnormalities provoked by exercise.

Fiber—the undigested portion of fruits, vegetables, and grains. The components of fiber are divided into those that are water soluble (pectins, gums, mucilages, and some hemicelluloses) and those that are insoluble in water (lignins, cellulose, and the remainder of the hemicelluloses).

Fibrocystic breast disease—usually painful, cystic swelling in the breast. The discomfort is usually worse before and during menstrual flow.

Fibromyalgia syndrome (FMS)—a syndrome characterized by a generalized deep muscular aching and associated with fatigue. The disorder is more common in women than men and may be associated with a sleep disturbance.

Fight/flight response—another term for the stress response, which occurs often unconsciously whenever the brain perceives a threat. When this happens, the body first tries to protect the vital organs.

Flatus—gas or air passed from the rectum.

Functional disorder—a disorder characterized by abnormal bodily function without a known, identifiable structural or biochemical abnormality.

Gallbladder—a saclike structure located under the liver that stores bile. Gallstones may form in the gallbladder, blocking the exit of bile and producing intense pain, usually in the upper abdomen.

Gastroenterologist—a physician with special training in the diagnosis and treatment of diseases affecting the digestive system.

Generalized anxiety disorder (GAD)—unrealistic nervousness often resulting in stomach trouble, insomnia, and other ills, and lasting more than six months. GAD and autonomic hyperactivity are different names for the same disorder.

Giardiasis—a parasitic infection of the intestinal tract, caused by the Giardia protozoa, which produces a diarrheal illness.

Gland—an organ that secretes a specific substance.

Glucose—a simple sugar, also called dextrose; the principal simple sugar in the human body and body fluids.

Glutamic acid—a protein used to produce the sodium salt MSG through a manufacturing process.

Gluten—a protein found in wheat and other grains.

H2 blocker—a class of medications that block the histamine2 receptors in the body. Most frequently, these medications are used to treat disorders that result from or are made worse by excessive acid secretions in the stomach (for example, peptic ulcer disease).

Helicobacter pylorus—a bacteria believed to cause inflammation and ulcers of the stomach.

Hemorrhoid—a mass of dilated veins around the rectum or anus.

Hepatic flexure syndrome—a pain syndrome produced when gas or air accumulates in the upper aspects of the colon on the right side, under the liver.

Hiatal hernia—protrusion of a portion of the stomach through the diaphragm into the chest.

Hydrogen breath test—a test used to determine lactose intolerance as well as other conditions. During the test, samples of expired air are analyzed for hydrogen content.

Hyperalgesia—the magnification of pain that frequently occurs with chronic pain disorders in which a person is very sensitive to changes in bodily sensations.

Hypoglycemia—an abnormally low level of sugar (glucose) in the blood. Symptoms include headache, rapid heart rate, sweating, nausea, mental confusion, and faint feeling.

Indigestion—failure of digestive function. Indigestion usually refers to acid indigestion (heartburn), which produces burning pains in the chest and may result from eating certain foods, eating too much, or eating too fast.

Inflammation—a tissue response to injury or destruction marked by redness, heat, and/or pain, among other symptoms. The injury may be produced by a variety of means, such as infection, excessive acid, excessive sunlight, or extremes of temperature.

Inflammatory bowel disease (IBD)—those disorders that involve inflammation of the intestinal tract and are often characterized by severe, sometimes bloody diarrhea, abdominal pain, and weight loss.

Insulin—the hormone produced by the pancreas gland that regulates the rate at which the body utilizes carbohydrates. An absolute or relative deficiency of insulin results in the disorder referred to as diabetes.

Internist—a physician specializing in the treatment of adult medical problems. Traditionally, internists have special training in the treatment of diseases that affect the internal organs. An internist is to an adult as a pediatrician is to a child.

Intestinal adhesion—an abnormal fibrous band that develops between internal organs, often after abdominal surgery.

Lactase—the enzyme that is deficient in the intestinal lining of patients with a lactose intolerance.

Lactase enzyme supplement—enzyme supplements that are obtained in liquid or tablet form to treat patients with lactose intolerance.

Lactose intolerance—an inability of the body to metabolize the complex carbohydrate lactose and the result of deficient amounts of lactase enzyme. Symptoms include cramping abdominal pain, diarrhea, bloating, belching, and excessive gas.

Laparotomy—surgery of the abdominal cavity.

Lipase—the enzyme that catalyzes the decomposition of fats into smaller subunits.

Lower esophageal sphincter—the one-way valve between the esophagus and the stomach that ordinarily prevents food from going back up or regurgitating into the esophagus.

Lower GI— See Barium enema.

Manning criteria—a set of criteria developed in 1978 by Dr. Manning and colleagues to help diagnose IBS, in which six common symptoms were noted.

Mastication—the chewing of food; the only voluntary aspect of digestion.

Metabolism—the sum total of the processes and reactions whereby the body utilizes the nutrients absorbed into the bloodstream after food has been digested.

Motility—ability to move spontaneously.

MSG—monosodium glutamate is a food additive used as a flavor enhancer in many packaged, processed, and frozen foods.

Mucin—a mixture of proteins that is the chief constituent of mucus.

Mucus—the free slime of the mucous membrane, composed of its secretion, mucin, and various salts and body cells.

Neurotransmitters—a chemical involved in the sending of nerve signals between nerves. The neurotransmitter serotonin is a major player in the motility of the gastrointestinal tract. There are various medications available that affect the nerve receivers of serotonin in an attempt to control IBS symptoms.

Nicotine—the substance found in tobacco products that may lead to indigestion, increased blood pressure, and constriction of blood vessels. It has also been linked to heart disease, lung cancer, and other diseases.

Nonulcer dyspepsia—burning "ulcerlike" abdominal pains in the absence of a demonstrable ulcer by X rays or endoscopy.

Obsessive-compulsive disorder—characterized by persistent, inflexible thoughts that lead to compulsive urges, such as the excessive preoccupation with details and strict standards in the completion of tasks.

Panic disorder—characterized by sudden attacks of intense fear, with physical symptoms that may include chest pain, palpitations or chills. Panic attacks are often associated with specific situations, such as airports or shopping centers.

Palpitation—a heartbeat that is unusually rapid, strong, or irregular.

Pancreas—a large gland located below and behind the stomach. It secretes insulin to help regulate the blood glucose and also secretes various enzymes that aid in the digestive process.

Parasympathetic nervous system—that branch of the autonomic nervous system that normally concerns itself with "energy-conserving" properties. Activation of the parasympathetic nervous system results in, among other things, decreased heart rate, decreased respiratory rate, and increased blood flow to the digestive organs. The major neurotransmitter of the parasympathetic nervous system is acetylcholine.

Peptic ulcer—a sore on the inner part of the stomach or duodenum, thought to result from excessive stomach acid or a breakdown of the mucosal lining of the stomach or duodenum.

Peristalsis—the wavelike progression or alternate contraction and relaxation of muscle fibers found in the alimentary tract that serves to propel the contents along.

Phobia—anxiety connected to an irrational fear of something specific such as speaking in public or a food.

Placebo—an inactive substance resembling a medication that may be given during experiments to determine psychological effects.

Premenstrual syndrome (PMS)—a syndrome characterized by mood changes, irritability, breast swelling and tenderness, abdominal cramps, and fluid retention that occurs 10 to 14 days before the onset of menstrual flow.

Primary-care physician—usually a family physician, internist, or pediatrician who provides preventive care and treats medical problems when they occur. The primary-care physician makes appropriate referrals to specialists when required.

Probiotics—healthy bacteria introduced into the colon to establish and maintain normal bowel flora, often prescribed to follow a course of antibiotics.

Proctalgia fugax—intense rectal pain occurring as the result of spasms of the muscles around the anus.

Protease—the enzyme responsible for breaking down proteins into their smaller constituent amino acids.

Purgative—a medicine that produces a purging effect and results in free evacuation of feces.

Radioallergosorbent test (RAST)—a blood test used to determine the presence of antibodies to various substances that may cause allergic reactions.

Radiologist—a medical doctor with specialized training and expertise in X ray procedures.

Rate of Perceived Exertion (RPE) Scale—a scale that is used when prescribing intensity of exercise and that correlates descriptive terms with numbers.

Rectum—the lowest portion of the large intestine, which stores feces until elimination.

Red flags—symptoms or conditions, such as fever, weight loss, and anemia, that suggest the existence of an alternative (other than IBS) or coexisting disease.

Reflux esophagitis—the regurgitation of acid stomach contents into the esophagus, which produces burning pains frequently referred to as heartburn or indigestion.

REM—rapid eye movement, one of two stages of normal sleep, with the other being non-rapid eye movement (NREM). NREM sleep is divided into four successively deeper stages, with stage four being the deepest. Dreaming takes place during REM sleep, while the fourth stage of NREM is the restorative stage of sleep.

Rheumatologist—a physician with special training in treating rheumatologic disease—those diseases that produce pain in the joints or muscles.

Rome II criteria—a set of criteria developed in 1999 by an international group of experts in the field of functional GI disorders that facilitates a diagnosis of IBS.

Satiety—the state occurring when one feels full or satisfied.

Side effect—a consequence other than that for which a medication is used, especially an adverse effect on another organ system.

Sigmoid exam (sigmoidoscopy)—direct examination of the interior of the sigmoid colon by the use of an endoscope.

Sitz bath—a warm water bath often used to treat conditions of the rectum or vagina. Enough warm water is placed in a tub to just cover the rectal or vaginal area.

Smooth muscle—sheets of muscle fibers found lining hollow structures in the body such as blood vessels, the intestines, bronchial breathing tubes, and the uterus.

Somatization—the use of physical symptoms for conscious or unconscious gain.

Spastic colon—the most frequently used synonym in the past for irritable bowel syndrome (IBS).

Spigelian hernia—a protrusion of the intestinal contents through a weak area in the lower, lateral abdominal wall, usually occurring in women after one or multiple pregnancies.

Splenic flexure syndrome—a pain syndrome produced when gas or air accumulates in the upper aspects of the colon on the left side under the spleen.

Stool specimen—fecal discharge from the bowel that is collected and submitted for laboratory evaluation.

Stress—a physical, chemical, or emotional development that causes strain and can lead to physical illness.

Sympathetic nervous system—that branch of the autonomic nervous system that is also commonly referred to as the "fight or flight" response. This branch of the autonomic nervous system prepares the body to meet a threat or challenge by, among other things, increasing heart rate, increasing respiratory rate, and increasing blood flow to muscles. The major neurotransmitter of the sympathetic nervous system is adrenalin.

Symptom—a recognizable change in a person's physical or mental state, which frequently brings the person to a physician's office.

Syndrome—a group of symptoms or signs that, occurring together, produce a pattern typical of a particular disorder.

Target pulse—the pulse rate that should be ideally maintained for a defined period of time to optimize an aerobic workout. It is usually obtained by subtracting your age from 220 and multiplying by 0.70. (Please refer to Chapter 8, "The Importance of Proper Exercise," for a more detailed discussion.)

TCAs—tricyclic antidepressants, a class of antidepressants often used in doses lower than those used for depression to treat the abdominal pain of IBS.

Ulcerative colitis—a form of inflammatory bowel disease that involves inflammation of the colon and produces ulcerations or sores. Symptoms consist of severe, sometimes bloody diarrhea, abdominal pain, and weight loss.

Ultrasound—the use of sound waves to produce images of structures within the abdomen.

Upper GI—an X ray examination of the esophagus, stomach, and duodenum. During this exam, barium (a chalky liquid) is ingested to contrast and outline the esophagus, stomach, and duodenum.

Urinalysis—analysis of urine as an aid in diagnosis.

Villi—the multitudinous fingerlike projections covering the surface of the inner lining of the intestines that are designed to increase the absorptive capabilities of the intestinal tract.

Index

References in italics refer to illustrations or other sidebars.

233

Dear Reader:

I hope you find this third edition of *IBS: A Doctors Plan for Chronic Digestive Troubles* helpful in your search for relief from the troublesome symptoms of IBS. I have received much personal gratification from the feedback received from readers of the first two editions. As IBS is usually a chronic and recurring concern, about which new information is constantly emerging, I have developed a web site www.ibsinformation.com to provide updates in this area.

Gerard L. Guillory, M.D.